PMS:
SOLVING THE PUZZLE

Sixteen Causes of PMS
& What to Do About It

Linaya Hahn

Foreword by Jordan Goetz, M.D.
Introduction by Allan Warshowsky, M.D.
With Comments for Therapists
by Maryann Troiani, Psy.D.

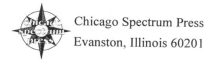

Chicago Spectrum Press
Evanston, Illinois 60201

PMS: SOLVING THE PUZZLE

© 1995 by Linaya Hahn

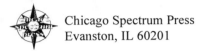 Chicago Spectrum Press
Evanston, IL 60201

READER PLEASE NOTE: The goal of this publication is to provide health care information for women of all ages who are interested in making informed decisions about their health. It is designed to heighten awareness of the latest research into premenstrual syndrome, but not to suggest diagnosis or treatment in individual cases.

The information in this book is meant to complement the advice and guidance of your physician. Since this publication is not a substitute for medical attention, the author and publisher cannot accept responsibility for application of this information to individual medical conditions, which in all instances should be managed by a physician.

Cover design by Dorothy Kavka
Page design and layout by Christopher Back
Graphs by Gene Mills
Illustrations by Art Henrikson

Printed in the U.S.A.

10 9 8 7 6 5 4 3 2 1

ISBN: 1-886094-15-2

To my parents
Who encouraged my curiosity

To my sister
Who stuck with me and taught me persistence

To my sons
Who taught me patience and gave me love and support

To my friends
Who taught me to believe in myself again

To all of them
They gave me love.

TABLE OF CONTENTS

FOREWORD

It's about time! Finally, a whole-person approach to a very difficult condition to deal with: PMS. The time-honored explanation of PMS as being "all in one's head" is dismissed, thank goodness, and replaced with "Yes, there is such a thing, and you're definitely not crazy."

PMS: Solving the Puzzle explodes the myth that PMS is a nebulous, untreatable condition—and goes one necessary step further: it outlines treatment options in a readable, informative fashion. The text is rooted in hard science, combining cutting edge research with time-tested remedies. It is quite complete, with thorough explanations and referencing. This book is *the* state-of-the-art text on PMS.

Science aside, there is another unique and important aspect to Linaya Hahn's book: its focus on the whole person. The holistic approach to medicine is coming back into favor here in the West: it has been an integral part of medicine in other cultures for centuries. *PMS: Solving the Puzzle* emphasizes that PMS has many factors in its etiology, the composition of which is as unique as every individual. The text concentrates on treating the person, not the disease. It shows people how to heal themselves, partly through self-empowerment, introspection, and healing from within. This approach is essential for a lasting treatment of PMS.

Ms. Hahn teaches us how PMS can be controlled in an empathetic, supportive manner. Her unique combination of genuine concern and solid information makes the readers' path to health clear, broad, and inviting. Truly, the journey through this book is refreshing and enlightening, giving hope and assurance to the PMS sufferer that all the pieces of the puzzle can fit together to make her a healthier woman, inside and out.

Jordan Goetz, M.D.
Former Chief of Internal Medicine
Vandenberg Air Force Base Hospital
Holistic Internal Medicine, San Luis Obispo, California

INTRODUCTION

It was the late 1960s. I was in medical school and becoming more and more disillusioned each day. Certainly there were enough doctors around. I just wasn't sure that they were really helping others. They were doing a lot of doctoring, but I didn't see much in the way of healing. Doctoring was often effective in changing a condition, but it didn't always seem to be in the best interest of the person being changed. Healing, on the other hand, while also involving change, uncovered the best natural aspects of the patient. With that realization I regarded myself as a healer-in-training rather than a doctor-in-training. Through the years, I've continued to evolve as a healer and to involve myself with like-minded individuals in order to facilitate my own growth.

It was through this involvement with healers that I met Linaya Hahn. Her caring connections with other people were immediately apparent to me. She was keenly interested in the positive growth of others. As an ongoing student, she was continuing her lifelong journey of education. Like a true healer and teacher, teaching what they need to learn, Linaya was healing herself of premenstrual syndrome (PMS) and learning about the puzzle that it represents to so many women. This book is the culmination of her work in the elucidation of PMS. There is a wealth of suggestions that the reader can adapt to her particular situation and begin to solve the enigma that PMS creates in her own life.

I became aware of PMS in the beginning of my private practice, about 20 years ago. PMS was becoming a popular and often-ridiculed diagnosis. It was generating stories and jokes like "I was premenstrual and he annoyed me, so I shot him...six times." These jokes, stories and anecdotes were not funny to me then as they are not now. At that time I found that by simply acknowledging women's premenstrual moods, thoughts and feelings, in conjunction with some dietary and nutritional changes, many women began to feel better. Adding some vitamin supplements increased the number who improved. Obviously, I had found some of the pieces of the PMS problem, but more needed to be uncovered. Many women and their families still suffered. I vividly remember telephone calls late in the evening, from husbands of my patients, begging me to do something, to give their wives anything to stop destructive episodes. But with the dearth of information, it was difficult to help.

PMS affects most, if not all, women in our society. Some have symptoms that are mild enough that they are not much of a problem. Others are probably too embarrassed or insecure to complain about how they feel. Some women suffer from what they and their doctors believe are either psychosomatic or otherwise unexplained symptoms that are part of the PMS complex. I would like to see this book turn on the light for these people. I strongly believe this book can heal.

The first step in healing is awareness. Awareness is needed for positive growth. Self-help involves self awareness and a willingness to accept responsibility. This book by Linaya Hahn is a powerful beginning toward that end. Women, and the others in their lives, who suffer from the seemingly inexplicable symptoms of PMS can begin to heal. The reasons for their premenstrual changes become clear. I want them to take the insights and observations from this book to an empathetic doctor or other health care provider and get the help they need to heal.

These are potentially positive and powerful times for women's lives. We are at a time, now, when we need women healed and whole. We need women to be aware of their uniqueness and their power. Female energy is needed to help all of us heal ourselves and our planet. This positive female energy comes from an awareness and a connection to what is purely female. Women must reconnect with pregnancy and childbirth, menses and menopause. Women need to integrate these essential aspects of their being in a healthy and constructive way. I applaud, praise, and highly recommend this book by Linaya Hahn as being an important step in that direction.

Allan Warshowsky, M.D.
Gynecologist
Lake Success, New York

Many of the people reading this book will undoubtedly be looking for help with their or a loved one's PMS. I hope this book will also be studied by the medical community, particularly by my colleagues in the mental health professions.

PMS is a problem that we as therapists need to take more seriously and become educated about. PMS makes life's challenges harder to deal with. It colors women's perception of the world. It blocks the energy they need to cope with their problems and it interferes with their life. Mental health professionals who attempt to treat their patients without considering possible physical complications like PMS are cheating their patients, denying them the best opportunity to get well.

One woman I worked with was constantly physically sick. No sooner had she recovered from one cold than she caught another. She had so little energy that she frequently couldn't get off the couch. Too tired to keep up with her friends or family, too weak to leave the house and get involved in her own life, her life was falling apart. Unsurprisingly, she soon grew depressed. She didn't respond to the approach prescribed by traditional medicine, antidepressant drugs.

Suspecting that her problem was at least partly physiological, we decided to concentrate on improving her physical health. We followed the regime described in *PMS: Solving the Puzzle*. She started to feel relief from her chronic illnesses. Once she began feeling better physically, she was able to see life and its options more clearly. It was as if she had been crawling, and suddenly she could walk upright. She had gained a new perspective on her problems. She became more productive. She started thinking more clearly and solving her problems. Even her husband observed physical changes as well as attitude changes in her. She is so energetic that he recently wondered, "How do you keep going?"

This kind of vibrant health is a wonderful end in itself. It is also an invaluable aid in effective psychotherapy. I urge mental health professionals to take a close look at their patients. Make sure they are healthy enough to tackle their problems effectively. It is ironic but true: sometimes the first step in helping a patient cope with psychological issues should be to help her overcome poor physical health.

The approach described in *PMS: Solving the Puzzle* works because it takes advantage of the interdependence between the mind and the body to achieve better overall health—the famous mind-body connection. In addition to thorough treatment of such familiar physiological tactics as eating better and exercising, the book has an excellent chapter on coping with stress. Ms. Hahn's approach is similar to that taken by Robert Atkins, M.D., although she concentrates on issues specific to women with PMS. Dr. Atkins reveals that the top two reasons why people seek psychiatric treatment are: 1) systemic Candidiasis and 2) chronic fatigue syndrome. Both Candidiasis (yeast infections) and fatigue are frequently linked to PMS, and both of them are addressed in *PMS: Solving the Puzzle*.

Once individuals overcome their physical roadblocks, then psychotherapy can help them resolve stressors and be fully healthy. *PMS: Solving the Puzzle* provides a wealth of information for professionals as well as the general public in achieving this goal.

Maryann Troiani, Psy.D.
Clinical Psychologist
Forest Psychcare Hospital
Des Plaines, Illinois

ACKNOWLEDGMENTS

My first acknowledgment must be to "my" women. I've become very protective of them and their feelings. They pushed me to find answers when they weren't feeling well, and once they were feeling better, they wanted to help other women feel healthy too. They wanted this information written in one place for all women to learn from.

Next I wish to acknowledge my son, Chris, and my sister, Sherrill, who read every sentence countless times and helped me make sense out of what I had written. The clarity of presentation is due in large part to them.

I would also like to thank my son, Greg, and my parents, who supported me every step of the way. Without them, this book would not be here.

Most of my information came from outstanding and generous doctors. First is Dr. Katharina Dalton, who insisted in the 1940s that PMS was real. Although I have identified additional causes of PMS, Dr. Dalton will always have my admiration for her uphill fight to bring attention to PMS.

JoAnn Friedrich, P.A., spent hours on the phone with me sharing her information about sleep and serotonin, the basis for classic PMS. Barbara Parry, M.D., taught me about light and its PMS connection. Jacob Liberman, O.D., Ph.D., and John Ott, Ph.D. (Hon.), gave me the answers about full spectrum light that I had been searching for. Dr. Iain Esslemont answered my questions about light in Australia.

Foremost among my recent mentors are Bob Anderson, M.D., preconference instructor for the American Holistic Medical Association. Alan Gaby, M.D., taught me about thyroid system malfunction and osteoporosis. John Lee, M.D., quickly sent me his important book, *Natural Progesterone*, when I was looking for his research.

Allan Warshowsky, M.D., gynecologist, believed this information needed to be compiled and published. He somehow found time to read the draft, suggest additions, and write a wonderful foreword. (Any errors that remain are, of course, mine.)

I am delighted to call Jordan Goetz, M.D., my friend. Besides checking for accuracy, he encouraged me when I got frustrated.

Maryann Troiani, Psy.D., insisted that therapists would benefit from recognition of many psychological challenges that are really physical in origin.

Gene Mills knew what the graphs would look like if he didn't help. His precision was essential.

Beth Russell, who fought PMS, Candida, and Hurricane Hugo at the same time, still found time to provide moral support. Thanks to Janet Jones, too, for her constant encouragement and support. We've learned a lot from each other.

Thanks go to Beryl Krejci for unearthing information linking Candida, thyroid, and progesterone. She is also a great proofreader. (We snuck in a few errors after she proofed the book, I'm sure.)

I would like to thank Rosemary Herhold and Mirra Rose for being with me when I needed them. I'm sure there are angels dancing on your shoulders. Thanks go to Dorothy Benish for researching lost items and to Pam Ryan, John Ross, Carol Stein, Carolyn Jackson, Ann Brazeal, Diane Breslow and Mary Shackle for proofreading. Thanks to Sue Mitchell, Lynn Bromm, and Sue Penrod for urging me to start this project long ago.

Art Henrikson added joy and laughter to my life when working on the book became a struggle. With his unique brand of magic, he translated my ideas into the marvelous pictures that brighten every chapter.

As you know by now, I did not write this book alone. "My" women, my family, doctors, therapists, nutritionists, and unseen forces guided me in this work. We all hope that you will benefit from our efforts.

Linaya Hahn
January 1995

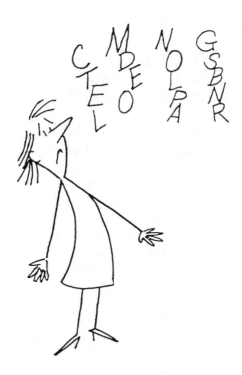

PMS IS A PUZZLE

PMS is a puzzle. Women and their doctors have had a difficult time trying to fill in the missing pieces. We try the latest approach discussed in the media, such as taking calcium or magnesium pills, going off caffeine, or increasing exercise, or we try something that worked for a friend. Unfortunately, we are often disappointed when that approach doesn't work for us. So we quit.

Some of us have learned from society that menstruation is a curse and expect to feel bad. Other women are aware that they are more inventive and creative before their periods.

Yet when the next outburst or bout of depression hits, we again resolve to be strong and not let PMS control our lives. Everyone is telling us to handle it. Other women can. Why can't we? We often feel that we'll never get through it.

In frustration, we wonder why doctors don't *do* something. Antidepressants, tranquilizers, and diuretics mask the symptoms,

1

but they don't eliminate them. It's good to be less depressed, tense, or bloated. But what is causing these symptoms in the first place? Can we correct the underlying problem and become fully healthy?

Doctors are trying to design a definitive study and to create laboratory tests that will help them select the proper treatment for PMS, but a conclusive ironclad study of premenstrual syndrome is nearly impossible to construct. Medical studies try to isolate one variable—such as cholesterol intake—and find out if changing that variable creates corresponding changes elsewhere—in heart attack rates, for example. There are so many environmental and hereditary factors that influence PMS, however, and so many different symptom patterns, that a study that took all of them into account would be impossibly cumbersome. The typical compromise is to control a manageable set of variables, such as birth control pill, antidepressant, and tranquilizer use, number of pregnancies, and hormone levels, but this approach ignores other possible causes, such as sleep patterns and antibiotic use.

PMS, by its very nature, is also very difficult to measure quantitatively. Depression, irritability, even physical symptoms like breast tenderness can't be measured as easily as blood pressure or cancer survival rates.

We will never find the cause of premenstrual syndrome because there isn't just one. There are many causes of PMS, many pieces of the puzzle. Addressing a single cause will help to some degree, but until all the pieces are in place, the symptoms will still occur.

I have had severe PMS. My PMS is now under control; in fact, most months I don't notice any PMS symptoms at all!

And I'm frustrated. Women with PMS should not have to hurt any longer. There are many effective new ways to control PMS, but it takes far too long for the latest research information on premenstrual syndrome to reach women and their doctors. That's why I wrote this book.

It is important to remember, especially with PMS, that every woman is different. In listening to women with PMS since the early 1980s, I've learned that no two have identical symptoms or patterns. Some experience devastating physical symptoms that control their lives; for others the psychological symptoms are the most overwhelming. This bewildering combination of symptoms and patterns is one of the reasons PMS is so confusing to the medical community.

I know from my personal and clinical experience that *women do not have to have PMS!* I feel better and more energetic today than I did in my mid-30s. Of the over 150 symptoms which are related to PMS, I've had most of them to some degree. I hope your experience is not as bad as mine was. Even if it is, there is hope. You *can* get over it.

The key to feeling better is to identify the pieces of your PMS puzzle and then take steps to put your health back together. Just as there is not just one cause, there is not just one answer. But there are answers!

Let's put your PMS puzzle together. Let's give your story a happy ending.

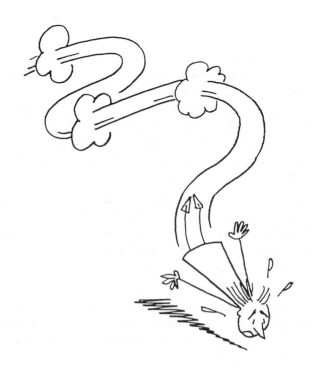

WHAT IS PMS?

PMS, or premenstrual syndrome, is defined as a medical problem characterized by a group of symptoms that appears before menstruation and disappears once menstruation actually starts. Over 150 symptoms have been found to be related to PMS. Although we hear most often about the psychological ones, such as irritability and depression, there are actually more physical symptoms, such as headaches, breast tenderness, and bloating. The physical symptoms alone can be devastating. PMS can affect every major system of the body: circulatory, digestive, immune, dermatological (skin), and nervous. It is very important that everyone understand that PMS is not a character defect. *A woman with PMS is not crazy.*

Researchers tell us that from ten to 90 percent of women have PMS at some time during their menstruating years. Ten to 90 percent? Can't researchers be more accurate? The problem is in defining premenstrual syndrome. We can include 90 percent if we include women with mild breast tenderness, fatigue, or headaches before their periods. Ten percent of women are severely affected. Although most women are aware of physical changes premenstrually, for most of us it is the psychological changes, such as depression or anger, which drive us to seek relief. If you think you have PMS, you're not alone.

Since PMS is so common, involving several million women in the United States alone and millions more worldwide, why wasn't it identified earlier? The delay in identification was a societal problem. Women didn't tell their doctors about their physical and psychological changes before their periods. And the doctors didn't ask how we felt, or assumed that with the normal physical changes in the body, there were bound to be disturbances, and told us there was nothing to be done. Well-meaning relatives and professionals often told us to get used to it. You may have been told that it was "all in your head."

As I've mentioned, there are no definitive laboratory tests which identify the causes of PMS, so the medical community, which relies heavily on tests, doesn't know how to approach it.

Many of us thought that female gynecologists, because they also experience menstrual cycles, would be more likely to under-stand women with PMS than their male counterparts would. This is not always the case. Like women who do not experience symp-toms during their own menstrual cycles, female gynecologists who don't have PMS sometimes have trouble relating to the experiences of those who do. Also, gynecological training focuses on female physiology, such as breast exams, Pap smears, pregnancies, and hysterectomies, often to the exclusion of related emotional factors.

If women mention anger, depression, or headaches before their periods, they may be referred to a psychologist, psychiatrist, or neurologist. This occurs not because the doctors don't care, but because these symptoms fall outside their area of expertise.

Doctors who did try to deal with these problems occasionally told the women to have their husbands take them out to dinner, or to have a more active sex life. Some were told to quit work, others to get a job, to have a baby, to wait until the kids left home, or to get married or divorced. Many women felt that these doctors were trivializing the symptoms.

Some women were told not to worry about the symptoms because "they will go away when your period comes." And often the symptoms do disappear completely, or at least become less severe, within a few days after the start of menstruation. The tragedy is that the symptoms come back each month.

The key to solving the PMS puzzle is to identify the possible causes and eliminate or correct them. To date, sixteen possible causes of PMS have been identified, and *none* of them means that you are crazy!

(Although psychiatrists can now diagnosis women with PMS as having Premenstrual Dysphoric Disorder, or PMDD, I'm not comfortable with a psychiatric label. The psychiatrists' position is that the diagnostic code enables them to obtain research funding to study the disorder. I'm concerned that the label may be used against women in cases of child custody or job qualification.)

There are only two things that you need to know about PMS:

- It is real.
- You don't have to have it.

I have a poster in my office with a quotation from Richard Bach's book, *Illusions*:

> *"You are never given a wish without also being given*
>
> *the power to make it come true.*
>
> *You may have to work for it, however."*

Let's get to work.

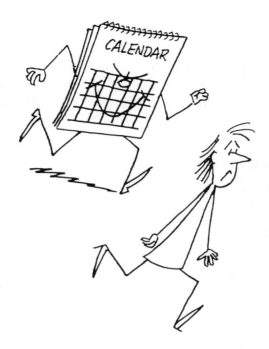

THE BASICS

When Does PMS Start?

Premenstrual syndrome can start two years before a girl begins her periods. It often lasts until menopause, when a woman's reproductive cycle stops. Even women who have had hysterectomies (sometimes called surgical menopause) can have PMS until they reach their natural age of menopause, which generally occurs in the early 50s.

PMS often starts after major hormonal changes, such as when a woman starts or stops birth control pills, after a pregnancy, or after a few missed periods. Tubal ligations or other abdominal surgeries, or IUD insertion or removal, may also mark the beginning of PMS or a worsening of its symptoms. Many women find that their symptoms increase in their mid-30s. Stress, either good or bad, may increase the symptoms. Some women are affected around menopause, although usually for a short time. All these events "insult," or influence, the

7

reproductive system. ("Insult" really is the word that doctors use!)

Let's look at the list of some of the most common events that knock our bodies out of equilibrium and start or worsen PMS. Put one check when you first noticed your PMS and two checks when it got worse.

_____ Puberty

_____ Going on or off birth control pills

_____ Inserting or removing an IUD

_____ Skipped periods (amenorrhea)

_____ Pregnancy

_____ Mid-30s

_____ Tubal ligation

_____ Hysterectomy

_____ Stress

_____ Menopause

What Happens During a Normal Cycle?

A cycle is the length of time from the beginning of one period to the beginning of the next. The first day of our flow is counted as the first day of the cycle, or day one. A "normal" cycle can be from 24-40 days in length. Most women average 28-29 days. That average, plus the convenience of a four-week calendar, is why birth control pills put us on a 28-day cycle.

The vast majority of women ovulate (produce an egg and can become pregnant) 14 days before their periods. (The word "ovulate" comes from the word "ova", or egg.) In a 28-day cycle, you probably ovulate on day 15. If you have a 24-day cycle, you may ovulate on day 11. A woman with a 40-day cycle would probably ovulate on day 27. At ovulation, many women experience a normal increase in vaginal secretion. In healthy women, this secretion is not a vaginal infection and does not itch, burn, or smell bad.

Menstrual flows (or periods or menses) normally range in length from three to ten days. Some women experience spotting before their flow starts or at the end of their flow. Some may have a little spotting at ovulation. Women tell me that when they become healthier, their menstrual flow becomes more efficient: it starts, it proceeds uneventfully, and it stops. Spotting often disappears, extremely heavy flows become lighter, and the length of the flow may decrease.

Incidentally, vaginal secretions change throughout the menstrual cycle. From our periods until ovulation, vaginal fluids increase daily, with the most fluid produced around ovulation. The fluid secreted at that time, which has an almost egg white consistency, keeps sperm alive as they travel up the Fallopian tube to fertilize the egg.

Does PMS Have a Pattern?

PMS has five distinct symptom patterns. The type of pattern helps to identify the cause. The first four patterns are varieties of what is commonly known as PMS. I call it classic PMS. The fifth pattern indicates a separate cause, atypical Candida albicans. PMS symptom patterns vary considerably between women, but each woman's pattern is usually consistent from month to month, although the severity of symptoms many change.

Pattern 1. Some women are affected for only a few days before their periods, although their symptoms may be severe.

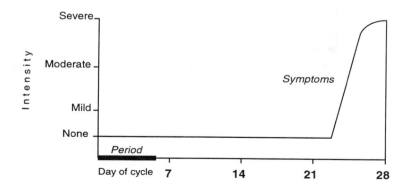

Pattern 2. Women in this group notice symptoms at ovulation and again just before their periods. This is a common teenage pattern. It may be even more confusing because of an irregular cycle length.

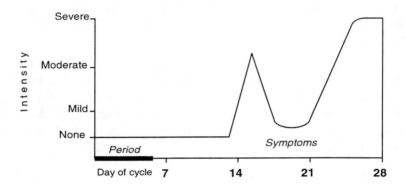

Pattern 3. These women have symptoms from ovulation until their periods come, for about two full weeks.

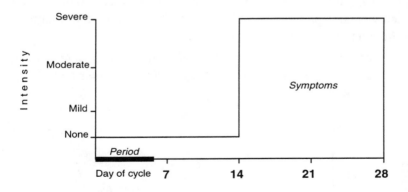

Pattern 4. Symptoms for this group seem to start before ovulation. These women actually ovulate a few days earlier than most, perhaps 16-17 days before their period rather than 14 days.[1]

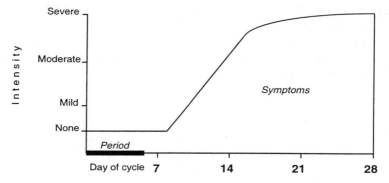

Pattern 5. Women in this last group follow one of the above patterns and have symptoms during their flow. PMS symptoms disappear when their periods start, but reappear a few days into the flow.

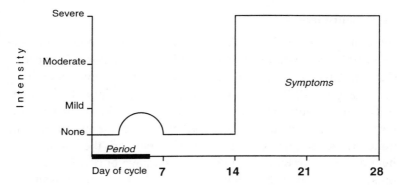

Over a longer span of time, a woman may notice both an increase in the number of days she is affected and an increase in the intensity of her symptoms. Some women have an even longer underlying pattern. They feel worse in the dark of winter and better in the summer sunlight. For others it is the reverse—they may have sufficient sun in the winter, but feel worse on humid, moldy summer days. A significant minority of women have a variation on the five standard patterns:

> *Recurring Pattern. The puzzle becomes even more confusing because some women feel bad every other month. Other women experience mild symptoms one month, moderate symptoms the next, and severe symptoms the third month. Then this larger pattern repeats itself.*

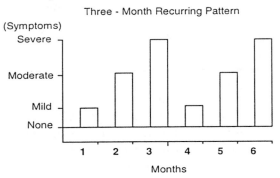

Three - Month Recurring Pattern

PMS Symptoms

Remember that I said that PMS has over 150 symptoms? Most of the symptoms are quite common and have many possible causes. Men can have aching muscles, fatigue, headache, even bloating, just like your PMS symptoms—but they certainly don't have PMS! I have included a list of 94 symptoms. You may wish to mark the ones you have. Each symptom may be absent, mild, moderate, severe, or extreme. Some women mark the majority of them as severe or extreme. Other women have only a few symptoms, but they may be quite severe. Still others don't want to mark any as severe. After all, they are coping, even though they feel terrible.

As you mark the list, be honest with yourself. You have nothing to gain by hiding a symptom or its severity. By acknowledging it, you can begin to find relief. Don't worry if you can't decide how severe it is. As one woman told me, "I can't decide how to mark 'indecision'."

Unfortunately, many women have had PMS for so long that they don't realize that they can feel any other way. If you can't decide whether a symptom is moderate or severe, circle both. Symptoms can fluctuate from month to month. By the way, husbands and friends frequently rate our symptoms worse than we do. Sometimes I think we don't want to admit to ourselves how badly we feel.

Incidentally, I had most of the following symptoms to some degree. If you do too, don't give up. I feel great now.

PMS SYMPTOM CHECKLIST

Please indicate whether your symptoms are absent (0), mild (1), moderate (2), severe (3), or extreme (4).

Absence from work/school 0	1	2	3	4
Abuse (verbal or physical) 0	1	2	3	4
Acne 0	1	2	3	4
Aggression 0	1	2	3	4
Alcohol (decreased tolerance) 0	1	2	3	4
Alcohol (increased consumption) 0	1	2	3	4
Allergies 0	1	2	3	4
Anger 0	1	2	3	4
Anxiety 0	1	2	3	4
Apathy 0	1	2	3	4
Appetite decrease 0	1	2	3	4
Arthritic-type pain 0	1	2	3	4
Asthma 0	1	2	3	4
Avoidance of social activities 0	1	2	3	4
Backache 0	1	2	3	4
Binges 0	1	2	3	4
Bloating 0	1	2	3	4
Breasts (swollen or tender) 0	1	2	3	4
Breathlessness or suffocation 0	1	2	3	4
Bruises easily 0	1	2	3	4
Circulatory problems 0	1	2	3	4
Cold sores 0	1	2	3	4
Confusion 0	1	2	3	4
Constipation 0	1	2	3	4
Cravings for salt 0	1	2	3	4
Cravings for sweets 0	1	2	3	4
Crying 0	1	2	3	4
Deodorant "failure" 0	1	2	3	4
Depression 0	1	2	3	4
Diarrhea 0	1	2	3	4
Disorientation 0	1	2	3	4

Dizziness 0	1	2	3	4
Drug abuse 0	1	2	3	4
Epileptic seizures 0	1	2	3	4
Excitability 0	1	2	3	4
Eye infections 0	1	2	3	4
Facial swelling 0	1	2	3	4
Fainting 0	1	2	3	4
Fatigue or lethargy 0	1	2	3	4
Genital herpes flare-ups 0	1	2	3	4
Glaucoma 0	1	2	3	4
Guilt feelings 0	1	2	3	4
Headaches (migraine) 0	1	2	3	4
Headaches (tension) 0	1	2	3	4
Heart pounding or irregularity 0	1	2	3	4
Hives 0	1	2	3	4
Hoarseness 0	1	2	3	4
Hot flashes or cold sweats 0	1	2	3	4
Hypoglycemia (low blood sugar)........... 0	1	2	3	4
Increased energy 0	1	2	3	4
Increased need for religion 0	1	2	3	4
Increased need to sleep 0	1	2	3	4
Increased sensitivity to light 0	1	2	3	4
Increased sensitivity to sound 0	1	2	3	4
Indecision 0	1	2	3	4
Intentional self-injury 0	1	2	3	4
Irritability 0	1	2	3	4
Irrationality 0	1	2	3	4
Joint pains 0	1	2	3	4
Leg heaviness 0	1	2	3	4
Loneliness 0	1	2	3	4
Loss of control (or fear of) 0	1	2	3	4
Mood swings 0	1	2	3	4
Muscle stiffness 0	1	2	3	4
Nausea or vomiting 0	1	2	3	4
Orderliness attack 0	1	2	3	4

Ovarian pain (sharp and one-sided) 0	1	2	3	4
Panic attacks 0	1	2	3	4
Paranoia or suspicion 0	1	2	3	4
Poor judgment 0	1	2	3	4
Poor coordination 0	1	2	3	4
Poor concentration 0	1	2	3	4
Restlessness 0	1	2	3	4
Ringing in ears 0	1	2	3	4
Self-confidence (lack of) 0	1	2	3	4
Self-esteem (lack of) 0	1	2	3	4
Sex drive (increase or decrease) 0	1	2	3	4
Shakiness 0	1	2	3	4
Sinus problems 0	1	2	3	4
Sleep disturbance 0	1	2	3	4
Sore throat 0	1	2	3	4
Spotting 0	1	2	3	4
Suicidal thoughts 0	1	2	3	4
Swollen hands, feet, ankles 0	1	2	3	4
Tension 0	1	2	3	4
Thirst 0	1	2	3	4
Tingling hands or feet 0	1	2	3	4
Urge to hit or throw 0	1	2	3	4
Urination (increased or decreased) 0	1	2	3	4
Vaginal itching 0	1	2	3	4
Varicose vein difficulties 0	1	2	3	4
Vision difficulties 0	1	2	3	4
Weight gain 0	1	2	3	4
Withdrawal from others 0	1	2	3	4

Other (please list)

_____	0	1	2	3	4
_____	0	1	2	3	4
_____	0	1	2	3	4
_____	0	1	2	3	4
_____	0	1	2	3	4

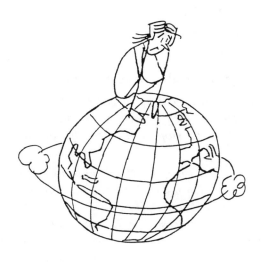

DOES ANYONE FEEL THE WAY I DO?

Your friends say they have PMS and complain of cramps or headaches for a day or two, or laughingly use PMS as an excuse to get something they want, like a sweater or being taken out to dinner. That is *not* the severity of PMS I'm talking about, and I don't like to hear PMS used as an excuse. Just as a person can be tired or exhausted, a woman can have mild or severe PMS.

You've checked the symptom list and probably marked a lot of them. You may have identified symptoms which you didn't know were related to PMS.

Here are some comments women have made to me about the symptoms on the list. I think you'll identify with many of them. Some comments made me laugh, some made me feel like crying.

Absence from work/school

"I can't skip work because I'm a full-time Mom, but I wish I could call in sick."

"I go to work, but I don't seem to get anything done. And when I do get something done, I'm likely to make more mistakes."

Abuse (verbal or physical) and aggression

"I can't believe what comes out of my mouth before my period! That's not me! I feel so bad afterwards, but I don't know how to stop it. I'm really an easy-going, happy person."

"During my good time, I tell the kids to clean up the cereal they spill. On my bad days, I find myself screaming, 'You stupid imbeciles! How could you be so clumsy? You're totally worthless! You'll never amount to anything!' I can't stop my mouth. Then they go down the driveway crying and I stand in the doorway crying. I don't even know why I exploded. I feel so guilty. They're really good kids. I've just destroyed their day and self-esteem as well as mine. How can they learn anything at school when they're so upset by such an awful, irrational mom? I feel so terrible."

Acne

"Why is my face breaking out now? The doctors call it adult onset acne, but don't know why. I want to hide. It's embarrassing."

Alcohol (decreased tolerance, yet increased consumption)

"During the first half of my cycle, I can drink a couple of drinks and not feel a change in behavior; during the last half, after two drinks I may be dancing on the table or sleeping under it!"

Anger

"I feel like Dr. Jekyll and Ms. Hyde."

Anxiety

"I get so jumpy I'm surprised my arms and legs don't fly off."

Apathy

"Nothing's right, but so what. I don't want to do anything about it."

Arthritic-type pain, backache

"I ache all over. I can hardly move. It hurts just to get out of bed in the morning. If this is what it feels like to be 35, I'll skip 65!"

Avoidance of social activities

"I've learned not to make any plans during the two weeks before my period because I'll try to get out of them. I tell my friends I'm busy, when what I'm really doing is sitting home and crying."

Binges

"How does five candy bars, five donuts (frosted) and a 1/2 gallon of ice cream sound?"

Bloating

"I feel like a blimp!"

"I'm miserable. I look like I'm five months pregnant."

Breasts (swollen or tender)

"It hurts to carry groceries."

"It hurts too much to be hugged. If you love me, wave from across the room. These are not to play with!"

"I have to have two different bra sizes. I even wear one to bed."

Confusion

"I'm always saying 'What?' Information seems to go in one ear and out the other. Yet on my good days, things are easy to understand."

"I feel like I have cotton for brains."

"I call myself 'Styrofoam-brain' because everything I hear just bounces off. Nothing sinks in."

Constipation

"I didn't know this was related to PMS but it is for me. I'm not constipated during the first half of the cycle."

Cravings for salt

"I didn't realize I had salt cravings. After all, I had a ham and cheese sandwich, pickles, and chips for lunch, with popcorn or pretzels for snacks."

"I used to fix popcorn 'for my kids' for about two weeks, then I'd stop. A couple of weeks later, I'd start fixing popcorn again. It took a while before I recognized the pattern and realized that I was really making the popcorn for myself."

Cravings for sweets

"Big time! One time I even pulled the car over to take a candy bar away from my daughter because she wouldn't share with me."

"I got up in the middle of the night to drive to an all night gas station to buy a chocolate candy bar!"

"I buy so much candy that I ask them to gift wrap it. But I don't give it away—as soon as I'm out of the parking lot, I open it and start eating."

Crying

"I cry all the time for no reason. Am I going crazy?"

"I'm just a puddle."

"I cried at Hallmark and telephone commercials on television."

"I cried at the Raid commercials when the bugs died!"

Depression

"I go to work and get a lot done. It's when I get home that I can't function."

Diarrhea

"Always—the week or so before my period."

"This hits when the flow starts."

Disorientation

"I got lost last night driving to a friend's house."

Drug Abuse

No one wanted to be quoted on this one!

Facial swelling

"My own sister said she wouldn't recognize me if she saw me on the street. My face was drawn and puffy, very pale and stressed-looking."

Fatigue or lethargy

"My kids were in school and I could do anything I wanted for a few hours. All I could do was go to bed. I didn't read, I didn't sleep, I didn't even roll over. I just lay there. On my normal days, I have lots of energy and am always busy and happy. What's happening? Please help me. I don't want to get attention by whimpering."

"I just feel totally drained."

Guilt feelings

"I hurt so many people so badly. I spend the good part of the cycle trying to make it up to them."

Hypoglycemia

"I get weak and dizzy and shaky all over. I can't concentrate. I've got to eat—now! But the blood tests don't show low blood sugar."

Increased energy

"The day before my period I start cleaning out closets or painting a room, then it feels like a chemical change comes over my body. I simply can't move. My husband gets mad at me for trying to do too much, but I know I could have finished the job if something hadn't switched inside me..."

Increased need for religion

"Dear God, please help me through this."

Increased need to sleep

"I'd like to sleep for two weeks!"

"I'm exhausted all day, but when I get to bed, I can't sleep. Sometimes I get to sleep, but I wake up several times a night and often have trouble getting back to sleep."

Increased sensitivity to sound

"Even the refrigerator bothers me. Sometimes when the refrigerator, freezer and furnace all stop at the same time during dinner I ask the whole family to stop eating and not move and just listen to the silence."

Indecision

"I can't decide how to mark that one!"

Intentional self-injury

"Sometimes the emotional pain is so bad I intentionally hurt myself because the physical pain takes my attention off the emotional pain."

Irritability

"Nobody can please me. I wear a frown all the time. The real me is easy to get along with. I don't know how people stand me."

Irrationality

"One time after a lovely dinner with my husband, he suggested we clean up the dishes since we were through eating. Something in me snapped. I grabbed the tablecloth with all the dishes on it and threw it in the garbage can! My poor husband. Do you know how foolish I felt the next day, digging plates and silverware and salt and pepper shakers out of the garbage?"

"Everybody, EVERYBODY, is WRONG. Even if they're right, I won't admit it."

Leg heaviness

"I work out all the time, but I can't do as much before my period."

Loneliness

"I felt lonely at my own birthday party. I felt people came because they felt they had to."

Loss of control (or fear of)

"I'm so afraid I'll hurt my kids. I never have, but I'm afraid I might."

Mood swings

"I don't even know how I'm going to feel and act in the afternoon. I'd like to have a body I can trust."

Orderliness attack

"My kids have to clean up their rooms NOW—or better yet, YESTERDAY! Sometimes I'm the tolerant mom with normal children, sometimes I'm the tyrant with

incredibly impossible, messy children. This really upsets me. Why can't I be consistent?"

Paranoia or suspicion

"I know my husband loves me. But at that time, if he's five minutes late coming home, I'm sure he's seeing someone else."

Poor judgment

"I hate to admit it, but last Friday before my period started, I filed for divorce, signed a lease on an apartment, and moved out. My period started Saturday." (P.S. They did get back together.)

Poor concentration

"On my good days I can understand the Encyclopedia Britannica; *on my bad days* Readers' Digest *is my level."*

*"I can't even do that—*Readers' Digest *is too hard! I just look at pictures."*

Self-confidence (lack of)

"My husband may tell me ten times that he loves me and I don't believe him because he didn't tell me eleven times. When I ask him if he loves me and he says, 'yes,' I don't believe him, either. I think that he only said it because I asked. Yet deep inside I know he does."

"It's hard to believe in yourself when you can't do anything right."

Self-esteem (lack of)

"I've got a wonderful group of friends and a long list of stuff I've done, but inside I feel that if someone really got to know me, they wouldn't like me."

"How can anyone stand to live with me? I don't even like to be with myself. Please help me."

Sex drive (increase or decrease)

"During the last two weeks of my cycle, I'd rather sit and watch anything on TV, yet I love my husband and have a good relationship with him. Bless him for understanding it's not him or me."

"My sex drive really increases just before my period. It's like, 'Honey, can you come home at lunch?'"

Shakiness

"It feels like there isn't a good nerve connection from my head through my neck to my fingers. I feel my hands shaking inside, but you can't see it when I hold them out."

Sinus problems or sore throats

"Always—just before my period."

Suicidal thoughts

"I know I won't do it, but it sounds like a good idea sometimes."

"I wish I could get on a plane that would never land."

"I hurt so badly emotionally, I wish I could go 'poof.' I don't really want to kill myself and I don't want to hurt anyone, but I don't want to live, either."

Swollen hands, feet, ankles

"My rings and shoes don't fit."

Tension

"I'm always jumpy the last few days before my period."

Urge to hit or throw

"Boy, would I like to let something fly! And I do sometimes."

Vaginal itching or burning

"I can't stand it. I've had infections for years. Nothing gets rid of them."

"I used to, but I haven't since the pregnancy. But that's when my PMS got more severe."

Weight gain

"I gain about four pounds every month, but I only lose about three and three-fourths."

"I can gain and lose ten to 15 pounds each cycle. I have to have two sets of clothes."

Withdrawal from others

"If I have plans, they usually get canceled. I'm to a point now that I generally just stay away from people because I'm afraid I'll say something awful. They probably don't want to be with me anyway."

None of these women want to hurt the people around them or to continue feeling miserable themselves. Did you hear the low self-esteem and despair in their voices? They're not crazy, just normal women who needed to find the missing pieces of their puzzle.

Many of you probably have many of these symptoms. They are common. Anyone can be depressed, have trouble sleeping, have vaginal infections, or digestive upsets. But is it PMS?

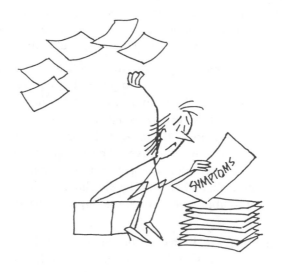

DO YOU HAVE PMS?

You are now aware that symptoms can start after major hormonal changes, you have seen the kinds of patterns the symptoms show, and you have read what the common PMS symptoms are and what some women say about those symptoms. But do *you* have PMS? We can begin to understand PMS and its causes when we check when the symptoms occur. Timing also helps us identify possible causes.

To date, routine laboratory tests cannot confirm PMS or identify its causes. So how is it diagnosed? You can do it yourself with a paper and pencil.

The Diagnosis

Write how you feel on a calendar as the symptoms happen and mark the date when your period begins. You need to see when your symptoms occur in relation to the period. If the symptoms cluster before your flow for two or three cycles, PMS is probably the cause. This is the only way to accurately diagnose PMS. You don't have to wait until your diagnosis is complete to start taking action, however. By following many of the suggestions in this book, you can begin to feel better *now*.

If the symptoms frequently appear on a certain day of the week, look at what is happening in your life then. Is it stress that appears once a week? What do you do on that day? Is it time to pay bills or hand in a report? What did you do or eat the day before? Did you sleep well the night before? Do the symptoms regularly show up on Mondays? These may be work-related symptoms. Or are symptoms worse on the weekend when stress, sleep, diet, caffeine, and alcohol levels change? Not everything is PMS. Other possible causes of the symptoms need to be ruled out.

I remember a call from a husband who telephoned for an appointment for his wife. He was taking the following week off work because he knew his wife wouldn't feel well then—it would be the week before her period. He wanted to help her and to take care of their son. His observations strongly pointed to PMS even before I met her.

Many times, the people who are close to us recognize PMS before we do. I'm not thinking about the insulting comments that are hurled at us in anger, "It's just your PMS talking!" I'm talking about the caring individual who notices tension in our voices before we are aware of it ourselves.

Confirming Your Diagnosis

You may wish to use the chart on the following page. Each vertical column can be a separate month. Choose three symptoms which bother you the most. Write them on the bottom of the chart. Then put the first letter of that symptom on the blank beside it. For example, for depression, put D. For bloating, put B.

I suggest you rate your symptoms as (1) mild, (2) moderate, or (3) severe. Then it becomes fun to watch the symptoms disappear. You CAN feel better!

Pattern 1 examples   MONTHS   *Pattern 2 examples*

	Oct.	Nov.	Dec.	Oct.	Nov.	Dec.
1			I^2		(P) Λ'	
2			I'		(P)	
3			$I^2 M'$			
4		I'	$I^- M^2 A'$			
5		I^2	$I^2 M' A^2$			
6	I'	$I' \quad A^2$	$I^3 M^3 A^2$			
7	I'	$I^2 M^2 A'$	$I^3 M^3 A^3$			
8	$I' M'$	$I^2 M^2 A^2$	(P) $\quad A^2$			
9	$I^2 M^2 A^2$	$I^3 M^3 A^3$	(P)			
10	$I' M^2 A^3$	$I^3 M^3 A^3$	(P)			$I^3 M^3 A^3$
11	$I^- M^3 A^3$	(P) $\quad A'$				$I^3 M^3 A^3$
12	$I^3 M^3 A^3$	(P)				$I^2 \quad A^2$
13	$I^3 M^3 A^3$	(P)			$I^3 M^3 A^3$	I'
14	(P) $\quad A'$				$I^3 M^3 A^3$	I'
15	(P)				$I' \quad A'$	I'
16	(P)			$I^3 M^3 A^3$	I'	I'
17	(P)			$I' M^2 A'$	I'	$I^2 \quad A'$
18				I'	I'	$I^2 M' A^3$
19				I'	I	$I^3 M^2 A^2$
20				I'	I^-	$I^2 M^2 A^2$
21				I'	$I' M' \Lambda'$	$I^2 M^2 A^3$
22				$I' M' A'$	$I' M' \Lambda^2$	$I^3 M^3 A^3$
23				$I' M' A^2$	$I' M' A^2$	(P) $I' M^3 A^2$
24				$I^2 M' A^2$	$I^2 M' A^2$	(P) M'
25				$I^2 M^2 A^2$	$I^2 M^3 A^3$	(P)
26				$I^3 M^3 A^2$	$I^3 M^3 A^3$	(P)
27				$I^3 M^3 A^3$	(P) $I' M^3 A'$	
28				$I^3 M^3 A^3$	(P) $M^2 A^2$	
29				$I^3 M^3 A^3$	(P) Λ'	
30				(P) $I' M^3 A'$	(P) $\quad A'$	
31		∿∿∿		(P) $M^2 A^2$	∿∿∿	

Symptom	Initial
1. Irritability	I
2. Migraine	M
3. Aching	A

Period = (P)

Symptom Intensity Code

Mild	1
Moderate	2
Severe	3

Example: Headaches = H

1	H-3	Severe headache
2	H-2	Moderate headache
3	(P)	Period

Pattern 3 examples.

Pattern 4 examples.

MONTHS

	Jan.	Feb.	March	June	July	August
1						
2						
3						
4						B^1
5						$B^1 F^1$
6					F^1	$B^1 F^2$
7					$B^1 F^1$	$S^1 B^1 F^2$
8				$S^1 B^2 F^1$	$B^1 F^2$	$S^1 B^2 F^2$
9				$S^1 B^1$	$S^1 B^1 F^1$	$S^1 B^2 F^2$
10				$S^1 B^1 F^1$	$S^1 B^1 F^1$	$S^2 B^2 F^1$
11		$S^3 B^3 F^3$	$S^3 B^3 F^3$	$B^2 F^2$	$S^1 B^1 F^2$	$S^1 B^2 F^2$
12		$S^3 B^3 F^3$	$S^3 B^3 F^3$	$B^1 F^1$	$S^3 B^2 F^3$	$S^1 B^2 F^2$
13		$S^3 B^3 F^3$	$S^3 B^3 F^3$	$S^2 B^1 F^1$	$S^2 B^1 F^1$	$S^2 B^2 F^2$
14	$S^3 B^3 F^3$	$S^3 B^3 F^3$	$S^2 B^2 F^2$	$S^2 B^2 F^2$	$S^2 B^1 F^2$	$S^2 B^2 F^3$
15	$S^3 B^3 F^3$	$S^3 B^3 F^3$	$S^3 B^2 F^2$	$S^2 B^2 F^2$	$S^3 B^3 F^3$	$S^3 B^3 F^3$
16	$S^3 B^3 F^3$	$S^3 B^2 F^1$	$S^2 B^2 F^2$	$S^2 B^1 F^2$	$S^2 B^2 F^2$	$S^3 B^3 F^3$
17	$S^3 B^3 F^3$	$S^2 B^2 F^2$	$S^2 B^2 F^2$	$S^2 B^3 F^2$	$S^2 B^3 F^3$	$S^3 B^3 F^3$
18	$S^3 B^2 F^2$	$S^2 B^2 F^2$	$S^3 B^3 F^3$	$S^2 B^3 F^2$	$S^3 B^3 F^3$	$S^3 B^3 F^3$
19	$S^2 B^2 F^2$	$S^2 B^3 F^2$	$S^3 B^3 F^3$	$S^3 B^3 F^1$	$S^3 B^3 F^3$	$S^3 B^2 F^3$
20	$S^2 B^2 F^2$	$S^3 B^3 F^3$	$S^3 B^3 F^3$	$S^2 B^3 F^2$	$S^3 B^3 F^3$	$S^2 B^3 F^3$
21	$S^2 B^2 F^3$	$S^3 B^3 F^3$	$S^3 B^3 F^3$	$S^3 B^3 F^3$	$S^3 B^2 F^3$	$S^3 B^3 F^3$
22	$S^3 B^3 F^3$	$S^3 B^3 F^3$	$S^3 B^3 F^3$	$S^3 B^1 F^3$	$S^3 B^1 F^1$	$S^3 B^3 F^3$
23	$S^3 B^3 F^3$	$S^3 B^3 F^3$	$S^3 B^3 F^3$	$S^1 B^3 F^3$	$S^3 B^2 F^3$	ⓟ B^1
24	$S^3 B^3 F^3$	$S^3 B^3 F^3$	$S^3 B^2 F^3$	$S^1 B^3 F^3$	$S^3 B^3 F^3$	ⓟ
25	$S^3 B^3 F^3$	ⓟ B^2	ⓟ B^1	$S^3 B^3 F^3$	$S^3 B^3 F^3$	ⓟ
26	$S^3 B^3 F^3$	ⓟ B^1	ⓟ	$S^3 B^3 F^3$	ⓟ F^1	
27	$S^3 B^3 F^3$	ⓟ	ⓟ	$S^3 B^2 F^2$	ⓟ	
28	ⓟ B^1	ⓟ	ⓟ	ⓟ B^1	ⓟ	
29	ⓟ			ⓟ		
30	ⓟ			ⓟ		
31	ⓟ					

Symptom	Initial	Symptom Intensity Code		Example: Headaches = H		
1. Sleeplessness	S	Mild	1	1	H-3	Severe headache
2. Breast Tenderness	B	Moderate	2	2	H-2	Moderate headache
3. Food Cravings	F	Severe	3	3	ⓟ	Period

Pattern 5 examples?

MONTHS

	July	August	Sept			
1	(P)	(P) D^3F^3	D^1F^2			
2	(P)	(P) D^-F^2				
3	(P)					
4	(P) $D^-M^-F^1$					
5	(P) D^2M^2					
6	(P) D^-M^-					
7						
8			$D^2M^2F^2$			
9			$D^2M^2F^2$			
10			$D^2M^3F^2$			
11		$D^2M^2F^2$	$D^3M^3F^3$			
12		$D^2M^2F^2$	$D^3M^2F^2$			
13		$D^2M^2F^2$	$D^2M^2F^2$			
14	$D^3M^3F^3$	$D^3M^2F^3$	$D^2M^2F^2$			
15	$D^3M^2F^2$	$D^3M^2F^2$	$D^2M^3F^2$			
16	$D^2M^3F^3$	$D^3M^2F^2$	$D^3M^3F^2$			
17	$D^3M^3F^3$	$D^3M^3F^3$	$D^2M^2F^1$			
18	$D^3M^3F^3$	$D^3M^3F^2$	$D^3M^3F^3$			
19	$D^2M^3F^3$	$D^3M^3F^3$	$D^3M^3F^3$			
20	$D^2M^3F^3$	$D^3M^3F^3$	$D^2M^3F^3$			
21	$D^3M^3F^3$	$D^3M^3F^3$	$D^3M^2F^3$			
22	$D^3M^3F^3$	$D^3M^3F^2$	$D^3M^2F^3$			
23	$D^2M^3F^3$	$D^3M^2F^3$	$D^3M^3F^3$			
24	$D^3M^3F^3$	$D^3M^3F^2$	$D^3M^2F^3$			
25	$D^3M^3F^3$	$D^3M^3F^3$	(P) D^1			
26	$D^3M^2F^3$	$D^3M^3F^3$	(P)			
27	$D^3M^3F^3$	(P) D^1	(P)			
28	$D^3M^3F^3$	(P)	(P) D^3M^3			
29	(P) D^1F^1	(P)	(P) D^2M^3			
30	(P)	(P) D^3M^3	(P)			
31	(P)	(P) D^3M^3	———			

	Symptom	Initial	Symptom Intensity Code		Example: Headaches = H		
1.	Depression	D	Mild	1	1	H-3	Severe headache
2.	Mood swings	M	Moderate	2	2	H-2	Moderate headache
3.	Fatigue	F	Severe	3	3	(P)	Period

31

MONTHS

1					
2					
3					
4					
5					
6					
7					
8					
9					
10					
11					
12					
13					
14					
15					
16					
17					
18					
19					
20					
21					
22					
23					
24					
25					
26					
27					
28					
29					
30					
31					

	Symptom	Initial	Symptom Intensity Code		Example: Headaches = H	
1.	_____	____	Mild	1	1	H-3	Severe headache
2.	_____	____	Moderate	2	2	H-2	Moderate headache
3.	_____	____	Severe	3	3	(P)	Period

MONTHS

1						
2						
3						
4						
5						
6						
7						
8						
9						
10						
11						
12						
13						
14						
15						
16						
17						
18						
19						
20						
21						
22						
23						
24						
25						
26						
27						
28						
29						
30						
31						

Symptom   Initial   Symptom Intensity Code   Example: Headaches = H

1. _____ ____ Mild 1
2. _____ ____ Moderate 2
3. _____ ____ Severe 3

1	H-3	Severe headache
2	H-2	Moderate headache
3	(P)	Period

You don't have to have specific symptoms, or a certain level of severity, to have PMS. If a woman feels tired, bloated, or a little down before her period but isn't bothered by it, it's technically still PMS. In other women the symptoms may be so severe that personal and professional relationships are affected. You do not have to be suicidal to have PMS, although you may feel that way occasionally. If you regularly get respiratory, vaginal, or bladder infections or digestive upsets before your period, your condition may also be PMS-related.

Some women's symptoms become severe again around days three to five or four to six of their periods. Although these symptoms are not *pre*-menstrual, this distress *is* related to the menstrual cycle and can be helped by many of the therapies used to control PMS. Pay careful attention to the chapter on Candida.

Still other women suffer from cramps, endometriosis, or pelvic inflammatory disease (PID). Unfortunately, a woman with premenstrual syndrome may also have these problems. These conditions are not PMS, although eliminating PMS may reduce cramps and endometriosis symptoms.

Severe cramps may indicate muscle tension, which can be helped by stretching exercises, or they may indicate Candida or endometriosis. (We'll discuss Candida in Chapter 14.) Very intense cramps suggest a high prostaglandin level. The body produces prostaglandins to tell the uterus to contract and expel the unfertilized uterine lining. In some women the uterine muscle contracts so strongly that it actually cuts off the blood supply to the uterus itself. The resulting muscle cramps may be as painful as a heart attack. These high prostaglandin levels can be countered by taking an antiprostaglandin, such as ibuprofen, starting two days before the flow starts.

Some women benefit from taking supplements that contain essential fatty acids such as gammalinolenic acid or GLA. GLA and DGLA (dihomo gammalinolenic acid) can be obtained from Evening Primrose Oil and omega-3 and omega-6 fatty acids. (Available at your local health food store, or see the Resource Appendix.) Studies have confirmed that women with PMS respond well to additional essential fatty acids.[1,2] Fatty acid supplementation is particularly good for women with cyclic breast tenderness or lumpiness. A shortage can lead to an apparent excess of the female hormone prolactin.[3] Prolactin produces changes in mood and in fluid metabolism which are similar to PMS. Body tissue may be abnormally sensitive to normal levels of prolactin when they are low in essential fatty acids.

Our bodies can convert the linoleic acid (LA) that some foods contain into the necessary GLA, but this process is inhibited by ingesting too much alcohol, cholesterol, margarine, and trans fatty acid, getting too little zinc, or producing too little insulin. It is also blocked by stress, certain viruses, chemical carcinogens, and ionized particles in the air (such as that produced by computer monitors).[4]

Acupressure, chiropractic, and osteopathic treatments are used successfully by many women with menstrual cramps. An excellent description of which acupressure points to hold is shown in the book *Premenstrual Syndrome Self-Help Book: A Guide to Feeling Good All Month,* by Susan Lark, M.D.[5]

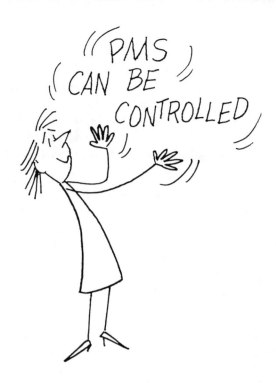

THE BEST NEWS

The good news about PMS is that it goes away; the bad news is that it comes back. The *best* news is that, once the cause is found, PMS can be controlled.

PMS does not disappear by itself. It may even gradually worsen with time. It was once called the "mid-thirties syndrome" because the severity of symptoms generally increases by that age. Many women who experience these changes think they are in early menopause (I hoped I was, but still had years to go) or are afraid that they are going crazy.

The biggest hurdle in relieving PMS is uncovering the cause or causes of PMS. To date, I have found sixteen possible causes of PMS. Which pieces of the puzzle will fall into place for you?

The causes are listed below, ranked from the easiest to the hardest to identify. Some corrections you can do for yourself; for others you will need a knowledgeable health care provider.

Sixteen Causes of Premenstrual Syndrome

1. Thyroid system malfunction
2. Caffeine
3. Poor diet, especially one with sugar and NutraSweet
4. Inadequate level of vitamins and minerals
5. Possible estrogen-progesterone imbalance
6. Sleep disorder (classic PMS)
7. Inadequate light
8. Atypical Candida albicans
9. Lack of exercise
10. Stress
11. Food allergies or sensitivities
12. Parasites
13. Environmental sensitivities
14. Mercury fillings
15. Exhausted adrenal glands
16. Unresolved physical or sexual abuse

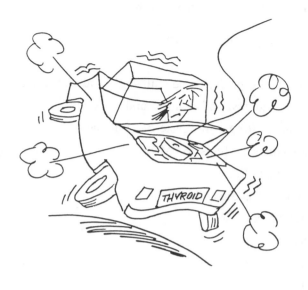

THYROID SYSTEM MALFUNCTION

I'm sure that many of you were surprised to see thyroid system malfunction as the first piece of the puzzle that needs to be ruled in or out. Early research indicated that one out of every six women with premenstrual syndrome has a thyroid problem. Some doctors have found that it is even more common than that. In the *New England Journal of Medicine*, Nora Brayshaw, M.D., reported that 51 out of 54 women with PMS had thyroid abnormalities as indicated by thyroid stimulating hormone (TSH) response.[1,2,3] Even with these dramatic numbers, many specialists believe the thyroid function test does not accurately measure the complete thyroid *system* function.

Thyroid system malfunction is best identified by symptoms. The thyroid is involved in several functions in the body, including menstruation, weight and body temperature (metabolism), hair loss, energy, depression, and immune system function. The pioneer in this field, Broda Barnes, M.D., Ph.D., tested 143 women with menstrual problems and found that 85 percent suffered from a poorly functioning thyroid system.[4] Thyroid system malfunction has also been linked to PMS due to its effect on immune system function and its connection to Candida albicans infections.[5,6] We'll discuss this in the chapter on Candida.

Menstrual cycle signs of thyroid system malfunction include:

- Early or late puberty (age nine or 17)
- Severe cramps
- Irregular periods
- Scant flow
- Bleeding between periods
- Heavy flow
- Some cases of infertility and miscarriage.[7]

One of the chief functions of the thyroid gland is to maintain normal metabolism and a normal body temperature. One of the most common symptoms of hypothyroidism ("low thyroid") is cold hands and feet, feeling cold "from the inside out." Many people with a poorly functioning thyroid system also have a low energy level and depression, although those symptoms can have many causes.[8,9]

Now we come to the frustrating part. Laboratory blood tests for thyroid hormone do not pick up all cases of a malfunctioning thyroid *system*.[10,11,12,13] Even when the thyroid stimulating hormone, or TSH, is also tested, many cases of thyroid system malfunction are missed. These people seem to exhibit cellular level tissue resistance to the thyroid hormone in their blood. This means that although normal amounts of thyroid hormone are present in their bloodstream, the individual cells do not receive sufficient amounts to work optimally.

(This cellular resistance to hormones is a familiar problem when testing for insulin sensitivity in diabetics, but resistance to thyroid hormone is a fairly recent discovery, one of which not all doctors are yet aware.)

In addition, we have recently learned that there are different types of thyroid receptors: one in the pituitary (which regulates thyroid production), and a different type in other areas of the body. With different types of receptors, the pituitary (brain) receptors may not know that other areas are low in thyroid hormone and so would not signal for an increase.

Fortunately, Dr. Barnes developed a simple, free, do-it-yourself test for thyroid function, known as the Barnes Basal Temperature Test.[14] A person who has a malfunctioning thyroid system often has a slow metabolism, which leads to a low body temperature. A simple way to check your thyroid is to get a glass mercury thermometer, shake it down and put it beside your bed at night. In the morning, with as little movement as possible, put it under your arm for seven to ten minutes and then note the temperature. This is generally your lowest temperature of the day. Write it on your chart. An underarm temperature reading is more accurate than an oral one because low-grade sinus infections can raise oral temperatures.

Take and record your temperature for several days when you first wake up. The normal axillary (underarm) temperature is 97.8° to 98.2° Fahrenheit. Some doctors say thyroid treatment is indicated when the temperature averages 97.4° or less.

Women should start taking their temperatures on day two of their menstrual cycle because of temperature fluctuations at ovulation and before their periods. If you've had a hysterectomy, start any day and continue the test for at least ten days. (Women still cycle after their uterus is removed until they reach their age for a natural menopause; they just don't have periods.)

If you have a relative with low thyroid function or suspect it from your own symptoms, I urge you to take your temperature, even if you have had a thyroid blood test in the normal range.

Temperature is a very good indicator of what is going on in the body. We appreciate the fact that our bodies strive to maintain a 98.6° temperature even when the external temperature varies from below freezing to very hot. The room temperature may be 70°, yet the body knows that for optimum health it should maintain an internal temperature of 98.6°. So it heats itself up 28.6°, to 98.6°. If it heats up an additional 1.4° to 100°, we say we have a fever. We ache, we are fatigued, we feel miserable. Couldn't a temperature that is 1.4° too low also cause symptoms?

Thyroid system malfunction may cause multiple enzyme dysfunction because enzymes function differently at different temperatures.[15] For example, most Siamese cats have silver-gray coats with darker hair on the feet and tips of the ears and tail. That is where their bodies are cooler. If a Siamese cat lives in a cold place, its hair will turn dark all over.

Before the thyroid blood test was developed, doctors treated thyroid system dysfunction by taking a careful medical and temperature history and noting symptoms which might respond to thyroid supplementation. Many doctors are returning to this approach to detect thyroid malfunction and possible PMS involvement. One medical saying is, "Treat the patient, not the blood tests."

Bear with me for the technical information. If a supplement is indicated, there are three prescription thyroid supplements. Cytomel, or T-3, is the most stimulating, but it is quickly metabolized, so the patient must take supplements more often. Synthroid, or T-4, the most popular prescription, is less stimulating but has a slower release and fewer side effects. It is converted by the body into T-3 and Reverse T-3. (Reverse T-3 is created by the body under stress. It does not stimulate the thyroid receptor sites, and it blocks the stimulating effect of T-3 and T-4. Reverse T-3, stress, fasting, illness, and cortisol all inhibit thyroid function.) Armour Thyroid, the best option, contains all three of the thyroid hormones: T-4, T-3, and di-iodo-tyrosine, called DIT.

Although medical textbooks state DIT is inactive, it *is* the maturation hormone for tadpoles. Since our bodies make it, logic assumes that it isn't inactive and is necessary. Perhaps we just don't know yet how it works. It wouldn't be the only chemical our bodies make that we don't fully understand. Since DIT is only made in the thyroid and the ovaries,[16] it makes sense to many doctors to supplement with Armour Thyroid (which contains the whole thyroid extract).

After you've taken your temperature for at least ten days, ask your doctor if it indicates a need for thyroid supplementation. If he or she is not familiar with this evolving area of medicine and is not yet comfortable with making a clinical diagnosis of thyroid system malfunction, you both may wish to read *Hypothyroidism: The Unsuspected Illness* by Broda Barnes, M.D., Ph.D.[17], or contact the Broda Barnes Research Foundation.[18] The Wright-Gaby Nutrition Foundation[19] also has valuable information for the general public and the medical community. Dr. Gaby's audio cassette, "Hypothyroidism: The Unsuspected Illness," and his letter to the *Journal of the American Medical Association* may be helpful in designing your program.[20,21] *Solved: the Riddle of Illness,* by Stephen Langer, M.D., describes the physical and emotional reactions of people with low thyroid.[22] Dr. Langer, too, has gotten quick and lasting results by identifying and treating poor thyroid system function.

The next question is, "How much is enough?" since the blood test may not be accurate for you. The gold standard in thyroid supplementation is, "How do you feel?" Again, "Treat the patient, not the blood tests."

I cannot close a chapter on thyroid and PMS without mentioning that undetected thyroid system malfunction has also been implicated in postpartum depression, or PPD.[23]

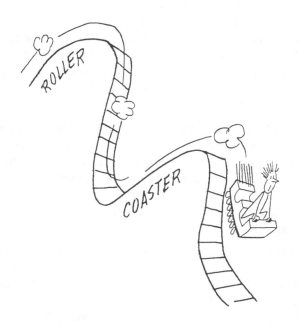

CAFFEINE

When I started trying to control my PMS, the first, and hardest, thing I did was to give up tea and cola-type drinks, like Coca-Cola and Pepsi, which contain caffeine. (I don't like coffee.) All the experts said to go off caffeine, but I didn't want to. I knew *I* wasn't addicted to caffeine. I only drank it for the flavor and the bubbles. I had a cola in the morning and again in the afternoon. I didn't crave sugar either. (A 12-ounce cola contains ten teaspoonfuls of sugar.[1]) I wasn't addicted to it. Wrong!

Since I felt so miserable before my period, I decided to go off caffeine for one cycle. I promised myself that if I didn't feel better, I could pick it up again after my period started. I quit cold turkey and had a terrible headache for three or four days, with cravings for the rest of the month. I really *was* addicted to the caffeine and sugar!

Imagine my irritation when I actually felt better before my period! But since I did, I decided to stay off caffeine for one more cycle. And I felt still better before my next period. So I stayed off a third cycle. I felt so much better by then that I couldn't even be tempted by chocolate, which also contains caffeine-like substances. Now I'll go thirsty before I'll drink something with caffeine in it.

How does caffeine affect us? Johns Hopkins researchers found that it blocks adenosine, a neurotransmitter which sends a message to the cells to slow down.[2] With the adenosine brake disengaged, the nerve receptors become hyperactive and hyperreceptive. If you're depressed, you'll feel more depressed; if you're irritable or anxious, you'll be more so. Whatever the symptom, caffeine magnifies it.

Researchers have found that caffeine can have effects ranging from increased alertness to jitteriness, anxiety, and sleeplessness.[3] Our nightly sleep patterns improve when we avoid caffeine completely, even in the morning. Caffeine can nullify the effect of a tranquilizer or a sleeping pill,[4] and classic PMS is a sleep-related disorder (more about that in Chapter 12).

Coffee is a major source of caffeine. A ten ounce mug of coffee made in a coffeemaker contains about 300 mg. Instant coffee contains less (132 mg), but enough to affect us. Most people don't have to worry about the amount of caffeine remaining in decaf coffee (approximately six milligrams in a mug), although some people find that the irritating oils in the coffee cause nausea, vomiting, diarrhea, and occasionally ulcers.[5]

The orange pekoe tea that we drink regularly in the United States contains 28-46 mgs of caffeine per cup, depending on how long it was brewed. (Longer brewing makes it stronger.) Green tea contains about one-fourth the caffeine of coffee.

Watch out for caffeine in chocolate and soft drinks, too. A small candy bar may contain 20 milligrams of caffeine. A 12-ounce can of Coca-Cola, Dr. Pepper, or Mountain Dew contains from 55-65 milligrams of caffeine. It wasn't worth it for me. You'll probably discover the same thing.

You could switch to decaf coffee, decaf tea, or herbal tea. Many women like hot or cold water with a slice of lemon. Try it! You'll probably find that you like it.

The following table shows the average amount of caffeine in different drinks:[6,7]

Coffee (10 oz. mug)

Drip (coffeemaker)	302 mg
Percolator	208 mg
Instant	132 mg
Decaffeinated	6 mg

Tea

Black (1 bag, 3 min. brew)	35-46 mg*
Green (1 bag, 3 min. brew)	20-33 mg*
Herbal/mint	0 mg

Carbonated drinks (12 oz. can)

Coca-Cola	65 mg
Mountain Dew	55 mg
Tab	49 mg
Pepsi-Cola	43 mg
Diet Rite	31 mg
7-Up, Sprite	0 mg

Other

NoDoz, Vivarin, Dexatrim, Aqua-Ban	200 mg
Excedrin	130 mg
Midol	65 mg
Anacin	64 mg
Baking chocolate, 1 oz.	35 mg
Milk chocolate, 1.5 oz.	9 mg
Hot cocoa (water mix, 6 oz. cup)	10 mg

*The variation reflects different amounts of tea in different brands' bags.

Be alert. Caffeine is also found in pain relievers, diuretics, cold remedies, and weight-control aids. Since I can't list all of them, read the label and avoid anything with caffeine.

Our bodies respond quickly to caffeine by releasing adrenalin, the fight-or-flight hormone. Sensing a crisis, our bodies dump extra insulin into the bloodstream. This insulin pushes blood sugar down. Surprisingly, our blood sugar is lower shortly after drinking a sugary soda than it was before. Blood vessels in the brain contract, while others in the body expand. The stomach secretes more acid and the kidneys more urine. We feel an energy spurt and then a drop. To pick ourselves up again, we frequently drink more coffee or soda. It's like being on an energy roller coaster.

Caffeine is often combined with sucrose in colas, coffee with sugar, and chocolate. Sucrose, the sugar found in most processed foods, is a complex sugar, formed by combining the simple sugars glucose and fructose. Most of the sugar enters the bloodstream (in the form of glucose) soon after ingestion, causing a rise in the blood sugar level. In response, insulin is then secreted by the pancreas to help the cells convert the blood sugar to usable energy. Sucrose increases stress on our bodies. It also weakens our immune systems for four to five hours after ingestion.[8]

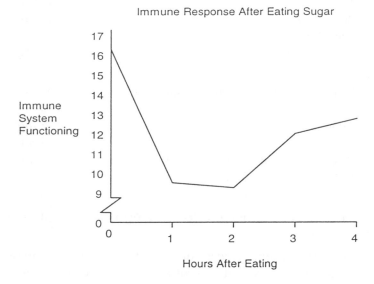

Immune Response After Eating Sugar

Our bodies run much better on slower, more even-burning fuels, like fructose, starch, and protein. Fructose, the type of sugar most often found in fruits and honey, is 50 percent sweeter than common refined sugar. Rather than spurting into the bloodstream and stressing our bodies, fructose is immediately trapped and stored in the liver. It is then very slowly converted into the kind of sugar our cells burn. Only then is it released into the blood. Fructose is released so gradually from the liver that it causes an even slower—and longer-lasting—rise in blood sugar than do many complex carbohydrates, such as breads, oatmeal, rice, potatoes, and peas.

This graph shows how the body uses different carbohydrates.[9] When caffeine is added, the body has a faster blood sugar rise and and sharper fall.

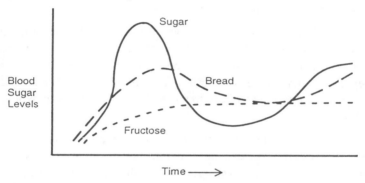

Our bodies convert all food, except fats, into blood sugar. Blood sugar gives us the energy to think and move. Our bodies don't need refined sugar to live. Refined sugar provides calories with no additional benefit. That's why sugar calories are called empty calories. When I write about sugar, I include table sugar, high fructose corn syrup, dextrose, maltose, honey, molasses, brown sugar, and maple syrup. High sugar (and high fat) snacks tend to edge out balanced meals. In 1976, soft drinks comprised 35 percent of all sugar consumption. These empty calories replace more healthful and less expensive foods. (Even diet soft drinks are no answer, because NutraSweet negatively affects the brain chemistry of women with classic PMS. See Chapter 12.)

Grains, vegetables, fruits, and protein are more nutritious than simple sugars because they are accompanied by vitamins, minerals, and fiber. Because they are digested more slowly, they give us moderately increased blood sugar and energy for a longer time. One study compared the body's reaction to table sugar (sucrose) and fruit sugar (fructose—in this case from raisins). Even though an equal number of calories were ingested, insulin levels increased 70 percent more after eating table sugar than after eating raisins.[10] The sugar was much harder on the body.

In case you haven't guessed it, my first suggestion is to reduce sugar and to go off caffeine, *gradually*. Cut your consumption by one-third for a few days, then another third for a few days, and then eliminate the final third. If you drink coffee, mix the regular with decaf. Even if you think you won't be able to wake up without it, give it a try. I think you'll be surprised in a few days and feel better before your period.

A study by Oregon State University supports the recommendation to go off caffeine.[11] Researchers examined the tea-drinking habits and PMS symptoms of 200 women in China. They found that those who drank from one-half to four cups of tea a day were twice as likely to suffer PMS symptoms as women who drank none.

If you need another incentive to eliminate caffeine from your diet, caffeine leaches calcium from your bones and contributes to osteoporosis. One study showed that one cup of coffee (approximately 150 mgs. caffeine) increased calcium loss by 30-50 mgs.[12] There is a direct relationship between the amount of caffeine ingested and bone loss. Another study of women ages 34-59 rated the relative risk for hip fracture almost three times higher in the group that drank the most caffeine compared to those who drank the least.[13] I know I won't grow taller as I age, but I don't want to "grow" shorter or break a hip, either.

Will gradually eliminating caffeine make a difference in *your* life? You'll be the first to know. Haven't you had PMS long enough? Aren't you a little curious to see if eliminating caffeine will help you? What have you got to lose, except some miserable symptoms?

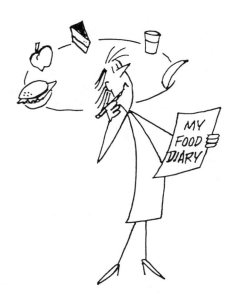

WHAT ABOUT DIET?

The next major part of the PMS puzzle involves the food we eat. When you analyze your diet, look at *why* you eat as well as *what* you eat. Do you eat because it's there? Or because it "called" you? Do you eat to satisfy cravings? Do you eat because it tastes good, or because it's good for you, or both? Maybe you're too busy to fix a "real meal," so you pick up whatever you see. Perhaps you eat when you're happy and excited? Or when you're lonely or bored? Maybe you eat something that makes you feel good right now, although you know you'll feel worse later.

Each of us could probably say yes to each of these questions at some point in our lives. Yet the statement "you are what you eat" couldn't be more true. We are kept alive by what we put in our mouths. Our diets help us build health, or drain our energy.

Do you skip meals in order not to gain weight? Please don't. You're stressing your body when you do. It's important to eat at least three times a day. And snacking can be good, too. (I'm snacking as I write.)

Aim for six half-meals a day. We wouldn't ask our families to go without a meal; treat yourself as well as you treat others. Cars don't run on empty; bodies don't either.

Diet, a good four-letter word, is simply what we eat. The way we ate when we were growing up still influences us. Did you always have dessert? Did you eat lots of vegetables? Maybe you had pizza every Friday night as a child. As an adult, it may not seem like Friday without pizza. Diets can be hard to change.

Lifetime eating habits may be difficult to change, but not impossible. A poor diet does not cause PMS, but for many reasons it can make symptoms worse. Foods which reduce PMS symptoms are not boring and tasteless; they may simply be different than what you are currently eating. Feeling well and having increased energy are such powerful rewards that those of us who no longer have PMS are not willing to return to our old habits. We like the increased energy that a quality diet gives us.

When you see something in the following list that you choose to add to your diet, great! When you listen to your body carefully, it gives you clues about what is good for you. You'll never know how much better you can feel until you try it.

It's easier to start a new eating plan when you view the changes as temporary. Changing your diet is not necessarily permanent, like having your appendix out. When you feel good again, you can add back the foods which you avoided during your recovery phase. If you reintroduce a particular food and you don't feel as good, you have a choice. Eliminate the food again and feel better, or eat the food and feel worse. Many have found that after several months of avoiding an offending food, they are able to reintroduce it occasionally with no problems.

The Harvard School of Public Health and the World Health Organization's European office propose the following Traditional Healthy Mediterranean Diet.[1] It's an update of the USDA pyramid. The idea is to build a strong base of foods from the bottom of the pyramid and to eat the foods at the top sparingly.

In comparison to the traditional American diet, the Mediterranean diet increases the amount of grains, fruits, vegetables, beans, and nuts. It recommends using olive oil for most of our fat and eating cheese and yogurt daily. It also recommends enjoying fish and poultry a few times a week and eating sweets, eggs, and red meat only rarely. This diet gives us more whole, unprocessed foods, foods that are nutrient- and fiber-rich. Mediterraneans, who follow this diet, have lower chronic disease rates and longer life expectancies.

You may actually eat *more* food on this diet because grains and vegetables don't contain as many calories per bite as sugar and oil. Better yet, people on the Mediterranean diet are likely to be less hungry, feel more energetic, and may well lose weight, because the slow-burning, high-fiber, nutritious foods it recommends provide a constant source of energy.

Although this plan draws as much as 40 percent of its calories from fat, about the current American average, the Mediterranean diet changes most of this fat to olive oil. Olive oil is a monounsaturated fat that is actually good for the heart and a reasonable source of vitamin E.

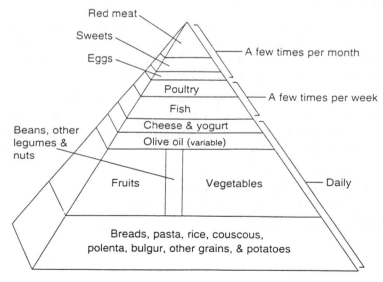

Traditional Healthy Mediterranean Diet

Now take another look at this pyramid, upside down. Doesn't it look like the traditional American diet, one that is about to topple over?

It is possible to cheat intelligently after you're well. By that, I mean eat a healthy diet and add just a little of the foods that might cause symptoms. Just don't indulge often. I remember going to a party and having a *taste* of three different cookies and giving the rest to a friend. Now that I eat what I want, I find that I choose foods that are good for me most of the time. I often hear women say they can't live without a specific food. Yet if they will avoid it for a short period of time, they often report that they never knew that they could be so energetic.

Foods that are good for women with PMS are good for everyone. You don't have to cook one meal for yourself and another for your family. Just because it's good for you doesn't mean that it tastes bad.

Small changes over weeks and months may be easier to accept and continue. For most people, radically changing your eating patterns in one week is stressful. The goal is to make better eating a lifelong habit.

When I decided to add brown rice to our family diet, I fixed it once a month because I was supposed to. Then I served it once every two weeks, then anytime. That way the whole family got used to the change gradually and learned to like it.

What we eat is an important piece of the PMS puzzle. A poor diet doesn't cause PMS but can make the symptoms worse. Small changes in the way you eat can have unexpectedly large results in how you feel.

So what do we eat? A fun rule to remember is, "Only eat foods that rot—just eat them before they rot!" Here are some foods that will turn all kinds of pretty colors if you forget them in the back of your refrigerator:

Foods To Eat

Vegetables

"Rainbow" diet—The deeper the color, the better:
Think dark green—broccoli, spinach, brussels sprouts
Think bright red/orange—beets, sweet potatoes, cabbage
Think onions and garlic

Salads

With lemon and olive oil dressing
Choice of spices

Fruit

Wide variety

Carbohydrates

Potatoes
Rice
Pasta
Whole grain cereals, breads, and crackers

Protein

Beans
Fish
Chicken and turkey
Beef, pork, and lamb
Cheese, yogurt, and eggs
Nuts

Oils

Olive oil

Drinks

Water (hot or cold—add lemon, if you wish)
Decaffeinated drinks

Foods To Avoid

Processed meats, such as hot dogs and lunch meat
Caffeinated drinks
Regular or diet soda
Sugar
NutraSweet, Equal, and aspartame

Smart Snacks

Remember those six half-meals a day? Snacks can be good for you. Snacking doesn't mean an automatic weight gain. Include health-promoting snacks in your daily nutritional goal. Our traditional American snacks of candy, soda, chips, and ice cream have a high sugar, fat, and salt content. These snacks tend to nudge out nutritious, full meals, plus they generally cost considerably more.[2] (Where else are we satisfied to spend more and get less?) You will probably feel better if you try some of the snacks below.

For a marvelous mid-afternoon pick-me-up, try:
> Fresh fruit
> Nuts
> Raw vegetables
> Sunflower seeds
> Popcorn
> Whole grain crackers and breads

For fun drinks, try:
> Herbal tea
> Water (hot or cold—it's good with lemon)
> Fruit and vegetable juices

I've found that meal preparation is easier when I'm not starving. I'm less likely to be too tired to cook or to snap at the people around me, and I don't pick up empty calories. So, start cooking or snacking before you're hungry!

Have you noticed the gradual appearance of organic fruit and vegetables in grocery stores? I recommend that you eat them whenever you can. One study tested five varieties of fruits and vegetables over a period of two years for twenty-two nutrients and four toxic elements. They found that "the organic pears, apples, potatoes, and wheat had, on average, over 90 percent more of the nutritional elements than similar commercial food."[3] A Rutgers University study found that organically grown tomatoes, for example, were over 500 percent higher in calcium, 1300 percent higher in magnesium, and an astonishing 193,000 percent higher in iron, when compared to nonorganic tomatoes.[4]

This is in addition to fewer pesticides. Organic produce is worth the extra cost.

Troubleshooting Your Diet

Some people don't feel well after they eat. They may grow tired or irritable or get a headache. They may become bloated or develop gas.

Tracking down a food culprit is easier if you keep a food diary. Write down what you eat, and then possible responses. Everyone knows that some people have allergic reactions immediately, getting a runny nose, a cough, a headache, or a swollen throat. Did you know that other people don't respond to offending foods for several hours or even three to four days later?

Use the following chart to see if you can discover a pattern between what you eat and how you feel. The pattern will be clear sometimes and confusing at other times. Include what you drink as well as what you eat.

You may wish to copy this page and jot down your diet for several days. Don't become discouraged if you see your eating patterns change before your period. That information is part of what we're trying to find out!

Diet Diary

Date _____   Day of Menstrual Cycle _____

        Food   Drinks   Symptoms

Breakfast

_____

_____

_____

_____

Snacks

_____

_____

Lunch

_____

_____

_____

_____

Snacks

_____

_____

Dinner

_____

_____

_____

_____

Snacks

_____

_____

_____

If your diet diary indicates that one specific food causes migraines, the puzzle is easy. (Not all migraines are associated with food sensitivities—some women's migraines are associated with their cycles. We will discuss that in Chapter 12.) However, a study from England reports that migraine sufferers react to an average of ten foods. The actual number ranged from one to 30. By eliminating those foods, 100 percent of the 60 patients, women and men, improved. 85 percent were headache-free. The aggregate number of headaches fell from 402 per month to six. That's impressive! Also, those with high blood pressure regained normal blood pressure on the elimination diet.[5]

British doctors and nutritionists have another tool which they use to combat migraines: an herb called feverfew. Several studies have shown that feverfew reduces the frequency and severity of migraines, as well as reducing nausea and vomiting.[6,7] Feverfew can be obtained from health food stores in either capsule or liquid form. It is most effective when taken as soon as a woman notices the characteristic aura that precedes the onset of a migraine.

Would it be worth it to change your diet? My experience suggests yes. Maybe the following outline will give you some ideas:

Symptom:	Irritability
Change:	Eliminate caffeine.
Why:	Caffeine makes nerves hypersensitive.
Symptom:	Breast swelling, tenderness
Change:	Eliminate caffeine and white wine. Add foods with vitamin E, such as dried beans, nuts, whole wheat, vegetables, and oils.
Why:	Vitamin E is a natural diuretic.
Symptom:	Hot flashes or toasty warm feeling
Change:	Eliminate hot drinks. Increase vitamin E.
Why:	Hot drinks require the body to get rid of the additional heat. Vitamin E reduces blood vessel dilation.

Symptom:	Fatigue
Change:	Eliminate sugar.
Why:	To stabilize blood sugar and eliminate Candida overgrowth.

Symptom:	Poor sleep
Change:	Eliminate caffeine. Increase complex carbohydrates, especially for dinner and evening snacks.
Why:	Caffeine even in the morning affects sleep at night. Carbohydrates such as vegetables and starches stabilize blood sugar.

A woman in my office recently asked, "Why didn't our mothers teach us this?" Much of the information on nutrition is fairly new, although it often indicates that we should eat more like our ancestors did—more whole foods, especially vegetables and grains, and less highly processed, sugary, and fatty foods. Our food also contains far more preservatives, artificial sweeteners, and sugar than years ago.

Our families can benefit from this information starting today. Our daughters need not have PMS, and our sons and husbands need not suffer with us. For more information, I recommend the books *Eat Right to Live Long*[8] and *Sugar Blues*.[9]

Many of us have accepted the idea that health means the absence of disease. I'd like you to think of health as more than not feeling bad. Health means feeling well, being resistant to disease, having energy, feeling alert. Given a chance, our bodies will fight to regain health; we only have to give them the opportunity. I plan to be healthy till I die. I hope you do, too.

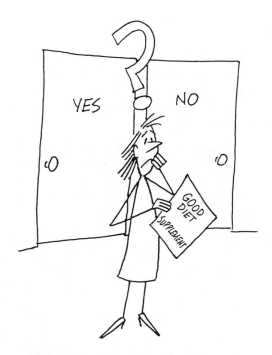

VITAMINS AND MINERALS – YES or NO?

Unfortunately, the story of the well-nourished American is a myth. We have plenty of food around us, but our choices are not always wise. Many of us are so busy that we rely on highly processed food or items from fast food restaurants. Others eat a calorie-restrictive diet to avoid weight gain. Did you know that people can suffer from undernutrition even though they are overweight?

The nutritional value of our food is affected not just by what foods we choose, but also by how it is stored, how it is transported, even how it is grown. Our food is often grown in mineral-deficient soil—ask any farmer.

Think of different plants which you have seen. Some are weak and spindly; others are vigorous and robust. The healthy ones received the right nutrients and light. People respond the same way. We, too, require essential nutrients. We can merely stay alive, or we can have lives full of energy and health.

We need 26 known essential nutrients from our food. Essential means that the body does not make them but must replace them daily from the food we eat. We must meet these essential requirements through carefully grown, fresh, varied food. We really are what we eat.

I have developed my own Broccoli Theory. I believe in eating quality foods like broccoli because many of the benefits of different plants are still being identified. And since I can't tell how my food was grown and transported by looking at it, I also take a multivitamin and mineral supplement.

We each have our own genetically determined nutritional requirements. Just as people come in different sizes, our vitamin and mineral needs also differ. Our nutritional requirements can vary by as much as 700 percent. These requirements vary according to age and emotional, biochemical, or physical stresses, as well as from individual to individual.[1] Biochemists and clinical nutritionists, who study how the body works on a cellular and molecular level, suggest an Optimum Daily Allowance (ODA) for optimum health.[2] The ODA is higher than the Recommended Daily Allowance, or RDA, which was set forty years ago by the U.S. Food and Nutrition Board. The RDA (the phrase is being changed to Daily Value, or DV) is the amount of nutrients necessary to prevent severe and potentially life-threatening diseases. Its recommendation on vitamin C, for example, is the amount needed to prevent scurvy. The RDA, or DV, does not tell us what is necessary for *optimum* health.

While it is possible to purchase vitamins and minerals at the grocery store or drug store, regular multivitamin formulas do not contain the high levels of nutrients which have been found helpful for women with PMS. I recommend you look for a "long list" formula, one with a long list of ingredients. Remember the 26 known essential nutrients? You can find good vitamin/mineral formulas in health food stores. Also, in the Resource Appendix I have listed places where you can order long list vitamins and minerals. Quality is essential. As my pharmacist says, the way the pill is formulated and even the way its ingredients are bound together influence the ability of the body to absorb it. To quote him directly, "Some pills go in looking like pills—and come out looking like pills!" You can guess how much was absorbed.

Some people are concerned about possible risks in taking high levels of vitamins and minerals. Statistics compiled by the National Capital Poison Center show that, in a typical year, several hundred Americans die from prescription drugs, but not one person dies from vitamin supplements.[3]

Be careful not to combine different pills with *very* high levels of *fat soluble* vitamins, such as A. The body does not excrete excesses of these vitamins efficiently. Beta carotene, which the body makes into vitamin A, can be taken in large quantities with no health risk. However, if the level of beta carotene is too high, your skin may turn a harmless yellow or orange. This disappears when beta carotene intake is reduced. Some women who have a thyroid system malfunction get yellow skin because their thyroid doesn't produce enough hormones to convert the beta carotene they eat into vitamin A. If you take more than one formula, check with a qualified health care provider to make sure your combined fat soluble vitamins are at a safe level.

Until recently, many doctors believed that eating a varied diet was enough for optimal nutrition, that people who took supplements just got expensive urine. They believed that people who got enough nutrients from their food to avoid deficiency disorders such as scurvy and rickets would not benefit from higher levels of nutrients.

The consensus is changing. More and more research indicates that taking vitamin and mineral supplements can make us healthier. Some compounds, such as antioxidants, may even retard the aging process. The most recent research indicates that people can have nutrient deficiencies in one organ even when the level of the nutrient is normal in the rest of the body. For example, a magnesium deficiency is often found in the heart muscle of people with heart disease, although the magnesium in their blood is at a normal level.[4] Elderly people with dementia often suffer from low levels of B_{12} in their brain tissue, although their blood levels are typically normal.[5] In such cases, blood tests for nutrient deficiencies won't find the problem.

Research is ongoing, but I think one fact is very revealing: most of the doctors and nutritional scientists who conduct the studies take vitamin and mineral supplements themselves right now.[6,7]

Nutrition specialists recommend taking a multivitamin/mineral three times a day with food rather than once a day to maximize absorption and interaction with the food we eat. Most of the benefit of each individual vitamin pill is metabolized within four to six hours.

A number of specialists believe that vitamin B_6 and magnesium can be particularly useful in targeting PMS symptoms. Recent studies indicate they are on to something:

Vitamin B_6

In a two-month randomized double-blind cross-over study of 48 women with PMS, 30 positive and six negative responses were recorded when 100 mg of B_6 was added daily. The placebo (a pill which looks identical but has no active ingredients) recorded ten positive and 20 negative responses. Symptoms included swollen breasts, abdomen, feet, and ankles, depression, irritability, fatigue, headaches, and stomach aches.[8]

Another study placed 434 women on either a placebo or 25 to 100 mg of B_6 for three months. Overall improvement was noted in 82 percent of the B_6 participants and 70 percent of the placebo group.[9]

A study reported in the British medical journal *Lancet* noted that 11 of 22 depressed women on birth control pills had a B_6 deficiency.[10]

Magnesium

The red blood cell magnesium level was significantly lower in 105 women with PMS than in 50 control women, although the serum blood levels were the same.[11]

A separate randomized double-blind placebo controlled study gave 32 women either 360 mg of magnesium three times a day or a placebo. Symptom levels fell significantly farther in the magnesium group at both the two- and four-month evaluations.[12]

Osteoporosis prevention, which has nothing to do with PMS, is also critically important to women. Osteoporosis literally means bones that are porous. Currently about a third of all postmenopausal women develop osteoporosis severe enough to get a fracture. That percentage nearly doubled between 1956 and 1983.[13]

Too many of us grow shorter or suffer from broken bones as we age because our bones are weak. Three major types of fractures occur: spine, wrist, and hip. A spinal fracture occurs when the front of one or more vertebrae becomes crushed, causing the spine to curve forward. This creates the hunched look we are so familiar with in older women. A wrist fracture can occur when we "break" a fall. Hip fractures are particularly dangerous: 20 percent of hip fracture victims die of complications within a year, and another 50 percent end up in a nursing home. Many others never return to full functioning after a break. Do I have your attention?

Osteoporosis can be prevented and even reversed. Bone is a living, changing tissue, just like the rest of our body. Ideally, we develop strong, resilient bones as we grow, but bone formation doesn't stop when we are teens. It goes through a continuous breakdown and rebuilding, or remodeling, process. As with PMS, it takes a comprehensive program to get the proper results.

It is no secret that women need calcium. Food and vitamin marketers, the media, and many doctors tell us that eating lots of calcium is the way to avoid osteoporosis. Many people assume that the goal is just to make sure their bones are loaded with calcium. It's not that simple. Even though bone is primarily calcium, we need more than calcium to create strong bones.

The trick is to have a complete program. Research indicates that the following nutrients are essential for healthy bones:

Magnesium has a positive influence on the type of calcium crystals present in bone.[14,15]

Boron reduces calcium and magnesium excretion.[16,17,18]

Zinc enhances vitamin D_3,[19] which bone-building cells require.[20] Low zinc levels have been found in people with osteoporosis[21] and with accelerated lower jaw bone loss.[22]

Copper deficiency reduces bone strength[23,24] and produces bone abnormalities in children.

Silicon is found at the building sites of growing bone.[25]

Manganese deficiency causes bones to be thinner than normal.[26,27]

Strontium appears to impart additional strength to bone and make them more resistant to resorption. It also appears to draw extra calcium into bones.[28] (Not all strontium is radioactive.)

Folic acid lowers harmful homocysteine levels (which come from high protein intake.)[29] Homocysteine can promote hardening of the arteries and osteoporosis if not detoxified.

Vitamin B_6 enhances the effectiveness of progesterone. Progesterone helps to rebuild bone.[30] B_6 also improves homocysteine metabolism and increases the production of structural proteins in bone.[30]

Vitamin C promotes the formation and cross-linking of these structural proteins.[32]

Vitamin D_3 is converted from cholesterol by sunshine (ultraviolet light). A deficiency causes "soft bones."[33]

Vitamin K is as important as calcium. Vitamin K helps to build the protein matrix where the calcium crystals form. Friendly intestinal bacteria make vitamin K for us unless an antibiotic destroys them.[34]

And, of course, bones need *calcium*. Calcium, like sodium, is usually found combined with other elements in molecules. Our bodies absorb calcium more easily from some of these compounds than from others. Some, like oyster shells, are very inexpensive but poorly absorbed; others are more expensive but much better absorbed (and therefore a better value). Microcrystalline hydroxyapatite (MCHC) is the best-absorbed calcium compound. MCHC contains most of the above micronutrients for excellent absorption. Microcrystalline hydroxyapatite has actually been shown to reimplant calcium in the bone.[35,36] Calcium citrate is also good, and somewhat cheaper. Calcium reimplantation is increased by adding magnesium and the trace element boron.[37,38]

In fact, researchers are now discovering that most women may need magnesium supplements even more than calcium supplements. Magnesium is crucial to a wide variety of metabolic processes, including the basic conversion of food to energy in every cell. It is also crucial to strong bones. Stress removes magnesium from the body.

Unfortunately, the typical American diet contains only 250 mg of magnesium a day, less than the Recommended Dietary Allowance of 350 mg a day, and far from the 600+ mg that is indicated for the Optimum Daily Allowance. The result is that many people have a significant magnesium deficiency. In addition to weaker bones, this can cause swollen breasts, abdomen, feet, and ankles. An Israeli study found that 16 of 19 osteoporotic women examined showed symptoms of magnesium deficiency. Each of the 16 had abnormal calcium crystals in their bones, while the three non-deficient women had healthy calcium deposits.[39] This may partly explain why some women with dense, calcium-rich bones still suffer osteoporotic fractures, while others with thinner bones escape.

Correcting these deficiencies can have a dramatic effect on strengthening the bones of women at risk for osteoporosis. Guy Abraham, M.D., examined 26 postmenopausal women. All ate well and were on hormone replacement therapy to slow their bone *loss*. (Bone density loss for early postmenopausal women averages 3 to 7 percent a year.) The 19 women who chose to take supplements (600 mg magnesium and 500 mg calcium) *increased* their bone density by an extraordinary average of *11 percent* in eight to nine months. The control group, on hormone replacement therapy but without calcium or magnesium supplementation, halted their bone loss, but they only gained 0.7 percent in density over the same period.[40]

When you choose supplements, be sure you are getting enough magnesium as well as calcium. Unfortunately, both take up a lot of room in a pill, so many of the one-a-day type vitamin/minerals don't contain much. Most of those that provide enough calcium and magnesium require you to take several— three to six—pills a day. Fortunately, microcrystalline hydroxyapatite (that special form of calcium), magnesium, and a good long list multivitamin/mineral, the kind which helps to control PMS, should contain enough of the above nutrients to help you avoid osteoporosis.

I also need to mention exercise. Our bodies respond to the stress of weight-bearing, low impact exercise by strengthening our bones.[41] Did you know that right-handed tennis players have stronger bones in their right arms than in their left? If you can, exercise outside. Full spectrum light causes cholesterol to be changed into vitamin D_3, which is essential for proper bone formation.[42,43]

Women's hormones have a big impact on the rate at which we lose (or gain) bone strength. That's why women are more affected by osteoporosis than men are. Most of us have heard that estrogen helps keep our bones healthy. Many postmenopausal women, whose estrogen levels are naturally low, take estrogen supplements for this reason. Recent research by John Lee, M.D., indicates that, while estrogen slows the rate of bone loss, we need progesterone to *build* strong bones.[44,45,46] Estrogen and calcium carbonate supplements (such as Tums) are not particularly helpful. We need natural progesterone and a well-absorbed calcium supplement to rebuild our bones and keep them resilient.

A complete osteoporosis prevention program should avoid foods that weaken bones. Eating large amounts of protein, especially red meat, increases calcium excretion.[47] Caffeine,[48] sugar,[49] phosphoric acid (found in all carbonated drinks),[50] and alcohol[51] increase calcium excretion in the urine. Colas, which contain caffeine, sugar, and phosphorus, are among the worst things you can drink if you're trying to prevent osteoporosis.

Smoking has also been implicated in bone loss.[52]

Let's recap. It is important to remember that supplements, no matter how good, can't stop bone loss alone. A diet with lots of green leafy vegetables, nuts, and whole grains will support your bones and you, literally. Progesterone and exercise outdoors or under full spectrum light are also important. Limiting soda, caffeine, alcohol, and stopping smoking helps you keep the calcium you have. If all of this seems too much to change at once, try making gradual changes. You don't have to change everything overnight, and don't worry about being perfect. "Intelligent cheating" is okay.

Will it be worth the effort? Dr. Lee's study showed that women following a similar program frequently exhibited an aver-age bone density *increase* of 15.4 percent, stabilizing at the levels seen in a healthy thirty-five-year-old.[53] The program is extremely effective and quite safe. A quality diet, nutritional supplement, progesterone, and exercise are not too much to do to keep us out of a wheelchair when we're older.

The definitive book on the subject is *Preventing and Revers-ing Osteoporosis* by Alan R. Gaby, M.D.[54]

Any review of how vitamins and minerals relate to women's health must mention folic acid. Folic acid, or folate, levels drop when a woman takes birth control pills and also during preg-nancy.[55] This can be very dangerous, since low levels of folic acid can cause spina bifida and brain damage in infants. Women who are pregnant or considering pregnancy, and women on birth control pills, should consider folic acid supplements.

And while we're off the subject of PMS, research shows that women with cervical dysplasia, a cellular disorder, are five times likelier to have low levels of folic acid. After taking ten mg of folic acid daily for three months, their biopsy results improved significantly.[56]

If the diet and vitamin/mineral information is confusing to you, look for a licensed nutritionist or doctor who practices nutri-tional medicine to help individualize your program. Laboratory tests can be run to assess your vitamin levels.

In addition to knowing what is good for my body, I always want to know why. If you are like me and want more information on how specific vitamins and minerals help women with PMS, there are excellent books on the subject. Check the Select Bibliography. If you can't find the supplements that you need, check the Resource Appendix for sources. Of course, these nutrients have many other effects on the body. Remember, supplements are recommended but are not a substitute for a quality diet—the Broccoli Theory again.

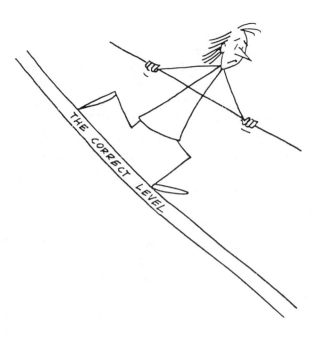

WHAT ABOUT PROGESTERONE?

So you don't have a thyroid problem (or you're on Armour Thyroid for it), you've cleaned up your diet, you're off caffeine, and you're taking a high quality vitamin/mineral. You've heard that progesterone supplementation helps some women. Could this be the last piece of *your* puzzle?

Progesterone and estrogen are the main female hormones of the menstrual cycle. Progesterone is produced in the body between ovulation and the start of the period, when PMS symptoms occur. Could it be that women with PMS don't make enough progesterone?

Progesterone calms the central nervous system and relieves many PMS symptoms. There are two forms of progesterone, natural and synthetic, with slightly different molecular structures. Our bodies make natural progesterone during the last half of each cycle and during pregnancy. Synthetic progesterone, found in birth control pills, Provera, and Depo-Provera, mimics natural progesterone but doesn't have quite the same effect. Synthetic progesterone can cause irritability, anxiety, depression, headaches, and insomnia. Dr. Katharina Dalton, the British gynecologist who first recognized PMS in the 1940s, has done ground-breaking research on it. She stresses the importance of natural progesterone supplements to treat PMS.[1]

Unfortunately, many well-meaning doctors prescribe synthetic progesterone in an effort to help women with PMS. Drug companies inform doctors about the (synthetic) progesterone products they make, but not about natural progesterone. Natural progesterone, an extract of wild yams, cannot be patented. Drug companies don't make it into pills or market it to us or to doctors because there is no profit incentive.

Natural progesterone supplements can be ordered only through a compounding pharmacist, who purchases natural progesterone in powder form and makes it into suppositories, suspensions, pills, creams, etc. (A compounding pharmacist has the additional training needed to formulate special prescriptions.) Unfortunately, the quality of these preparations varies.

Finding the correct level of natural progesterone for each woman is difficult and time-consuming. Six variables must be controlled for maximum effectiveness. A woman needs to start on the correct day of her cycle (ideally, two days before ovulation—whenever that occurs in the cycle), and then stop on the correct day (to allow the period to come). She must have the correct dosage level and the correct form of progesterone (vaginal or rectal suppositories, liquid suspensions, injections, pills, creams, or tablets to hold under the tongue), made by a pharmacy which can compound a high quality product, and she needs to take it at the correct time of day. Then she only gets one chance a month to get it right. You can see why good results are difficult to achieve.

Surprisingly, in spite of the fact that natural progesterone is helpful to many women, research has shown no correlation between PMS and progesterone levels.[2] Women with high *and* low levels of progesterone in their bodies can have PMS.

Many doctors prescribe progesterone for PMS, so I think a chapter on this treatment is in order. I have found that natural progesterone treatment, while helpful, does not completely solve the puzzle. For many women, myself included, natural progesterone supplements help reduce many symptoms, but do not eliminate insomnia, headaches, or food cravings.

I personally used vaginal progesterone suppositories four times a day, 17 days a cycle, for five years. It was terribly messy, but it gave me my life back. I was emotionally stable while on progesterone and could work to educate women about PMS. But although I no longer had headaches or food cravings, my insomnia remained.

I also noticed that some women experienced symptoms during their periods, when they should have been symptom-free. The body does not produce or require progesterone during menses and does not need supplementation at that time. These women could take progesterone during their periods to stop the symptoms, but then their periods would also stop. Obviously, progesterone did not complete the puzzle for these women.

A woman's complex, approximately 28-day cycle is produced by interaction between her brain and her reproductive organs. A period does not start until progesterone drops to a certain level. (That's why we don't have periods during pregnancies. Progesterone may rise as much as forty times higher during pregnancy than during the last half of each cycle.)[3,4]

To suppress symptoms which may occur during the flow, some women take progesterone for several additional days. This delays or slows down the menstrual flow, but it does not affect the natural rhythm of their *brain* chemistry. As a result, these women can no longer tell where they are in their cycle by noting when their period starts. Their brain thinks it is on the same old cycle, while their ovaries, etc., have had their cycle lengthened artificially. This becomes a real problem in subsequent months, as they try to figure out what day they should start taking progesterone again. Should a woman resume taking her progesterone on the fourteenth day after her (artificially delayed) period finally comes, when her ovaries expect it? Or should she resume taking the progesterone on the fourteenth day after her period would have come normally, when her brain and pituitary gland expect it? As the months go on, the timing can become even more out of balance.

Some women may be told to stop progesterone on day 28, even though their bodies operate on a 32-day cycle. Their symptoms may be more intense than usual after they stop.

Although I successfully regulated the timing of my cycles after 15 months, it was a very frustrating process. I can now teach someone how to regulate their cycle in a few months, but it is still frustrating and difficult.

There is no question that progesterone is important. If you are still interested in progesterone, an interesting study that used progesterone homeopathically (in minute quantities) was published in *Obstetrics and Gynecology*.[5] Other women find relief by using a cream which contains the extract of wild yam. (See the Resource Appendix for sources.) However, in my observation, there are several other important pieces of the PMS puzzle which, when identified and corrected, alleviate more symptoms.

While I was taking natural progesterone, I read an article about sleep and PMS. As I thought about my own sleep patterns, I realized that during the two weeks before my period my sleep pattern was still disturbed. I could go to sleep around 11:00 PM, but I awoke at 2:00 AM, and at 3:30 AM, and at 5:00 AM, or was awake for one and one-half to three hours. Then I was ready to sleep till 9:00 AM—but I had to struggle out of bed at 6:30 AM to go to work and get the kids ready for school. I was functioning, but exhausted.

When I awoke during the night, I frequently felt I had to urinate, but often it was such a small amount that it didn't seem worth the trip. So I tried staying in bed, telling myself that I had developed a bad habit. That didn't work either. I fell asleep again more quickly if I got up. I stopped drinking liquids after 7:00 PM. I still woke up. I exercised earlier in the day. I still woke up. Sometimes I woke up just to turn over. I always seemed to wake up facing the light from the clock radio. But *only* during the two weeks before my period.

I decided to look into sleep and PMS.

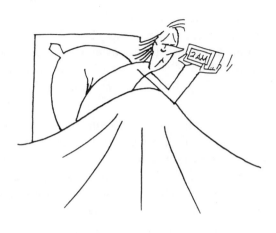

SLEEP

In the spring of 1986 I read about the work of JoAnn Cutler Friedrich, P.A. from Stanford University. She had had severe PMS and was not able to obtain relief with diet, exercise, or progesterone treatment. As she tells the story, she met with six women with PMS to find a common thread in their PMS experiences. What had happened to all of them in their twenties, their teens, or their pre-teen years that might have a PMS connection? Suddenly, someone said laughingly, "I know what I *didn't* do! I didn't go to slumber parties. I was a child bedwetter."

All six of them had been! Ms. Friedrich quickly called a seventh woman with PMS: she, too, had been a child bedwetter. Bedwetting normally affects only 3-4 percent of girls. She later said that if even one of them had not been a child bedwetter, she would have stopped her research into sleep and PMS.

As an adult, Ms. Friedrich slept 12-14 hours a night before her period and still woke up tired, crabby, and depressed. So she looked into sleep patterns as a possible common denominator for PMS. She found a definite correlation between sleep disturbances, brain neurotransmitters (messengers), and PMS.[1,2]

My sleep experience was just the opposite. I was not a child bedwetter, and instead of sleeping 12-14 hours a night, as she did, I had great difficulty staying asleep. She slept too much and I couldn't stay asleep. She was a child bedwetter and I was not. But we both had sleep disorders. I flew to San Francisco to meet with her.

Our business lunch lasted six hours. Ms. Friedrich identified PMS as a sleep disorder. How could that be? Wasn't PMS a hormone imbalance best controlled by exercise and dietary restrictions? Yet I was taking high levels of natural progesterone, exercising, and eating well, and I still wasn't healthy. I was waking two to three times a night. I kept asking questions.

The idea that a sleep disorder might be at the root of the problem intrigued me. If a person, man, woman, or child, doesn't sleep well, he or she may become irritable, depressed, or have trouble concentrating. It sounded suspiciously like PMS.

A sleep disorder is indicated by deep sleep, light sleep, or sleep disturbances. Sleep disturbances may show up as difficulty in going to sleep, nightmares, sleepwalking, talking in one's sleep, awakening during the night to go to the bathroom, or grinding one's teeth during sleep.

Sleep is controlled mainly by the neurotransmitter melatonin.[3,4] A neurotransmitter carries messages from one nerve cell to another. Melatonin is produced in the brain at night and when we are in dark, or dimly lit, areas. In sunshine or bright light, melatonin changes to serotonin, another neurotransmitter. People with high levels of serotonin feel alert and confident. Low serotonin levels have been linked to impulsiveness, aggression, and depression. Other research correlates low prolactin levels with low serotonin levels in the brain.[5]

Melatonin suppresses ovulation in women (and sperm production in men). Serotonin/melatonin levels must drop to allow ovulation to occur.[6] And that's when PMS symptoms start. Maybe *this* was the root of the PMS!

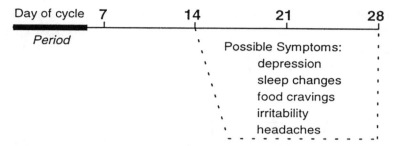

Serotonin drops to allow ovulation to occur.

Sleep patterns tend to run in families. You may have inherited a tendency for low serotonin/melatonin. There is a connection between low serotonin/melatonin and depression,[7,8] alcohol abuse, migraines, and sugar cravings.

According to a Swedish study which Jon Franklin reported in *Molecules of the Mind*, people have an 18 percent genetic risk for alcohol abuse if they have parents who abuse alcohol. That's close to the 25 percent incidence of Mendel's Law of Inheritance of Recessive Genes which governs whether we get blue eyes or brown eyes. The Swedish study noted that the sons of alcoholics may become alcoholics, but the daughters may have "ghost pains" whose cause is difficult to identify.[9] That sounded like PMS to me. A nurse I was working with at the time mentioned that a study showed that 75 percent of alcoholics have low serotonin levels.

But my parents and grandparents weren't alcoholics. My maternal grandmother had migraines, though. I looked into migraines and learned that a serotonin drop occurs when migraines start. And my mother has a mild sleep disorder: she grinds her teeth in her sleep. Did my PMS have a genetic tie-in?

Let's look at how we sleep. There are five stages of sleep which recur in 70-90 minute cycles throughout the night. The fifth stage, called REM (Rapid Eye Movement) sleep or dreaming, increases in length with each cycle. The longer REM periods which occur after several hours of continuous sleep seem to be the most beneficial. If your sleep is interrupted, your sleep patterns restart at the first cycle of the night. If you sleep too deeply and don't spend much time in the REM stage, you miss the effective dreaming or problem solving part of sleep. Sleep is not completely understood yet, but we do know that REM sleep is essential to functioning well.

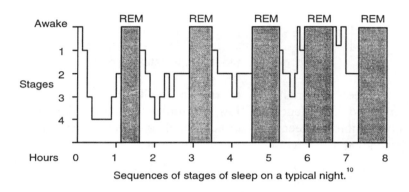

Sequences of stages of sleep on a typical night.[10]

Serotonin/melatonin brain chemistry is the same in women and men—until ovulation. Then, as I mentioned, these levels drop in women to allow ovulation to occur. Often that is when PMS symptoms begin, approximately fourteen days before the period begins. Is it possible that the normal serotonin drop at ovulation causes the symptoms of classic PMS? A study done at UCLA in 1987 confirms this.[11] Women who have classic PMS may have a genetic risk factor which is triggered by high stress. (See Chapter Three on The Basics.)

But some women have symptoms more than fourteen days before their periods. The *British Journal of Obstetrics and Gynaecology* notes that some women ovulate more than 14 days before their periods, even 16-17 days before their periods.[12] Remember, serotonin drops to allow ovulation to occur. Are the women who ovulate early the ones with low serotonin during the first half of their cycles? Medically speaking, these women have a longer than usual luteal phase (last part) in their menstrual cycles. (See Chapter Three, Pattern Four.)

Using ovulation prediction kits, I found that I was ovulating 17 days before my period! That was the same number of days that I needed progesterone to feel relatively well. Since progesterone helps to calm the central nervous system, I felt much better. But progesterone does not solve problems related to sleep disorders, headaches, or food cravings. We were treating my symptoms, not the cause.

I was afraid to go off natural progesterone. After all, I did feel better. For six months I procrastinated. But Ms. Friedrich challenged me to go off progesterone and take L-tryptophan, an amino acid which indirectly boosts serotonin levels.

The first month on tryptophan I ovulated 16 days before my period. The next month it was 15 days prior. The third month I ovulated 14 days before my period, just as I was supposed to. And my symptoms disappeared just as fast. I was delighted and astounded! I slept through the night and was happy and productive all day. Studies show that my experience is typical.[12]

How did that happen?[13,14] Our bodies make serotonin from tryptophan, an essential amino acid, or protein. "Essential" means that it must be replaced daily; the body does not make it from other foods. Fortunately, tryptophan occurs naturally in many foods, including turkey, milk, potatoes, eggs, fish, cheese, and soybeans.

Getting tryptophan into the brain is quite involved, but when there, it always results in increased serotonin.[15] Tryptophan must compete with phenylalanine, another amino acid, to cross the blood/brain barrier. Although essential to life, tryptophan is one of the least efficient amino acids in crossing the protective blood/brain barrier (the filter which protects the brain from bacterial infections, viral infections, and pollutants). When less tryptophan gets into the brain, serotonin levels are lowered.[16]

When serotonin is low, the brain starts a complex series of events to elevate its level of tryptophan. An insulin surge is needed to get the tryptophan into the brain. This may be noticed as a craving for sugar, pasta, bread, or alcohol. These carbohydrates quickly become blood sugar. The higher blood sugar triggers an insulin surge. This insulin surge has two effects:

it sends most of the other amino acids out of the bloodstream and into the muscles, and it helps tryptophan cross the blood-brain barrier.[17] Only phenylalanine, the other neutral amino acid, remains in the blood stream to compete with tryptophan to get into the brain.

A complication may occur here. NutraSweet and Equal, the trade names for aspartame, are made from phenylalanine, the only amino acid which competes with tryptophan for transport space.[18] Some people who consume products that contain phenylalanine report symptoms such as depression, irritability, sugar cravings, poor sleep patterns, or headaches, all common PMS symptoms. I recommend that all women with classic PMS stay off these products. (Note: G. D. Searle's patent on aspartame, the generic name for NutraSweet, recently expired, so products are appearing that contain aspartame but don't have the NutraSweet or Equal logo. Read the label and avoid everything containing aspartame.)

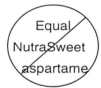 compete with tryptophan to cross into brain

I looked up all the entries about serotonin in a medical text, Harrison's *Principles of Internal Medicine.* It said that a "certain amount" of sodium is necessary to keep serotonin active in each cell.[19] Perhaps too little sodium leads to salt cravings. Was that why I ate potato chips and popcorn on my "bad" days and didn't on my "good" days? This may explain why many women with PMS crave salt before their periods. Their bodies may be trying to regulate their serotonin levels.

Vitamin B_6 is frequently recommended for PMS. I wanted to know why. I found out that vitamin B_6 is necessary to convert tryptophan to serotonin.[20] Another piece of the puzzle popped into place.

There is another way to support the body's use of tryptophan. When it enters the body, tryptophan can either become serotonin or niacinamide, vitamin B_3. So, to support the metabolic pathway of tryptophan, the diet may be supplemented with niacinamide. When the body has enough niacinamide, more tryptophan can become serotonin.[21,22]

(NOTE: Niacinamide is different from niacin. Niacin is used to lower cholesterol and may cause dangerous side effects. It must be monitored carefully by a physician. Niacinamide does not lower cholesterol and may be taken safely at higher levels. Niacinamide may help with sleep.)

At this point, light became one of the puzzle pieces. Light is needed for melatonin to be converted to serotonin.[23] Almost all of us, men, women, and children, feel better on sunny days, but I'm getting ahead of my story. More about light in the next chapter.

The following chart shows the pieces which must be in place for tryptophan to become serotonin or niacinamide. Carbohydrates activate the transport system which carries it into the brain. Sodium keeps serotonin active in each cell. Vitamin B_6 and light help in the conversion.

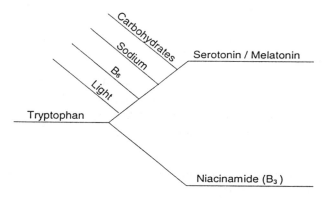

Before November 1989 women with PMS often reduced their symptoms by supplementing their diet with L-tryptophan. Tragically, four batches of contaminated tryptophan reached the market that month, and the FDA quickly and correctly pulled it off the market.[24] In some people the contaminated tryptophan caused a fatal hypersensitivity reaction called eosinophilia myalgia syndrome, or EMS. Unfortunately, on the supposition that tryptophan itself, not a contaminant, caused the problem, the FDA has not allowed it back on the market. It has since been shown that one manufacturer in Japan made a manufacturing error and allowed a bacterial contaminant to infect the four batches.[25,26] The problem has been fully identified[27] and the error that led to its production eliminated, but tryptophan remains unavailable in the U.S. It is still available and successfully used in other countries around the world.

(In fact, during the crisis, one doctor, Russell Jaffe, successfully treated EMS with uncontaminated tryptophan, along with two other supplements. He achieved complete remission of symptoms and a normalization of eosinophil (white blood cell) count in five weeks.[28])

People whom tryptophan helped, including women with PMS and people with migraine, sleep, alcohol, and drug problems, can no longer get it. Many of those people are put on Prozac and other serotonin-affecting drugs. Unfortunately, those drugs can have unpleasant side effects.

Women with the low serotonin levels of classic PMS can still be helped in spite of the FDA ban. Tryptophan is abundant in milk, turkey, and other food. Remember the adage that drinking milk at bedtime will help you sleep?

Stop a moment and picture Thanksgiving day. After a lot of turkey (which contains tryptophan) and sweet desserts, many people fall asleep during the football games on television. Is it only because of overeating and a change in schedule? I don't think so.

The foods highest in tryptophan and lowest in competing amino acids are potatoes, egg whites, and mustard greens. Other tryptophan-rich foods include cheese, fish, soybeans, cashews, millet, barley, cauliflower, wheat bran, lima beans, spinach, Brazil nuts, sunflower seeds, squid, scallops, clams, and oysters. You may wish to increase these foods in your diet.[29,30]

Sleep quality can be improved by two additional means. One way is to take melatonin. This is particularly effective for those who have trouble going to sleep.[31] Another sleep aid is valerian root. One study reported that people taking it went to sleep much more easily; another reported improved sleep in 89 percent of subjects, with 44 percent reporting perfect sleep, which was significantly better than the control group.[32,33,34]

I could sleep well again. My search for the cause of classic PMS was complete. Or was it? What about light?

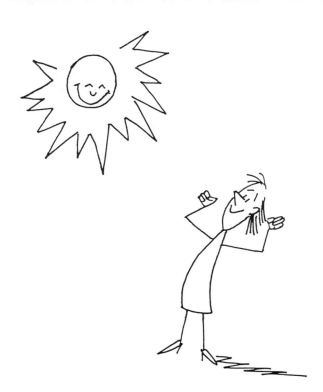

THE LIGHT CONNECTION

"Truly the light is sweet
And a pleasant thing it is for the eyes to behold the sun."

Ecclesiastes 11:7

"You light up my life."

People have known about the importance of light for ages. Children all over the world draw suns in their pictures to indicate happiness. We talk about getting a "bright idea." Our celebrities "bask in the light." We want to live on the "sunny side of the street." Poets remind us that in spring a young man's (or woman's) "fancy turns to thoughts of love" when the sun comes back.

Many of us notice that people are happier and more energetic on a sunny day. Think of a long stretch of cloudy weather and then remember people's responses when the sun breaks through the clouds. We smile more easily and accomplish more with less effort. Light affects both our moods and how clearly we think.

I first became involved with light in 1989. I was presenting a paper, *Multidisciplinary Assessment of PMS*,[1] at the annual meeting of the Dalton Society, an international physician-based organization for PMS research and education. While there I met Barbara Parry, M.D., from the University of California, San Diego, who was speaking on women and depression, specifically targeting PMS and light.

Dr. Parry, a psychiatrist, had previously done research on Seasonal Affective Disorder, or SAD, at the National Institute of Mental Health. SAD, identified in the early 1980s, is a pattern of mood and physical changes that has been linked to light,[2] to tryptophan,[3] and to melatonin.[4]

Imagine my excitement when Dr. Parry established a correlation between PMS and light! Her research with light fit my information about the serotonin drop at ovulation. She had identified a southern California woman who had PMS in the winter, but not in the summer. By putting the woman in front of bright lights, Dr. Parry found that her patient's PMS symptoms disappeared![5]

Basic research links PMS and winter SAD to low light exposure when there is weaker sunlight and fewer daylight hours. The weather is colder and people tend to spend more time indoors. The farther you live from the equator, the more seriously you may be affected. Near the equator, where sunlight is more constant and people spend more time outdoors, SAD and light-related classic PMS are less common and less severe. It is no coincidence that Alaska, Norway, and Sweden have some of the highest suicide rates in the world in the winter.

Typically, people with SAD become depressed each winter as the light fades.[6] These individuals may also gain weight, become anxious and irritable, oversleep, withdraw socially, or lose interest in sex. Many describe it as hibernation. Children generally react to the imperfect light by becoming irritable. They say they pick fights and don't know why.[7]

These symptoms sound like classic PMS to me. Classic PMS is similar to SAD except that PMS comes and goes monthly, not annually. Many women with PMS report that their symptoms decrease during the summer when they spend more time outdoors.

What is the connection between light and PMS? Light is the switch that raises our serotonin levels.[7,8,9,10] Serotonin and melatonin, two vital neurotransmitters, carry messages between nerves. Serotonin helps us feel calm, alert, and happy during the day. Melatonin is produced in the dark and helps us sleep deeply, which is why we sleep better in a dark room. When we get up in the morning and light enters our eyes, our brain stops producing melatonin and starts producing serotonin.[11,12,13] If we don't get enough light, or enough of the right kind of light, we may not fully wake during the day. We may not sleep as well either.

High melatonin

High serotonin

As you read in the previous chapter, serotonin drops to allow ovulation to occur. For some women, it falls low enough to cause symptoms of PMS. Then when their periods start and serotonin returns to its higher level, the symptoms disappear.[14]

So classic PMS is linked to light as well as serotonin. It really is physical in origin. **Classic PMS is caused by correctable irregularities in the normal brain chemistry changes that accompany ovulation. It is not a hormonal disorder.** We are not imagining things and we are not crazy! These changes happen in every woman; perhaps serotonin and melatonin fall lower in some women than in others, or perhaps some women are more sensitive to the drop.

Many of us are aware that we feel better on sunny days. That is when the body's level of serotonin is highest. When melatonin is high, we feel like sleeping or hibernating. We may eat as if we're getting ready to hibernate, too!

When serotonin is low, the brain signals a need for more serotonin, which we often interpret as a need to eat something, especially carbohydrates or sugar. Trying to satisfy the brain's call for increased serotonin is one of the reasons why many of us gain weight in the winter.

The amount of sunlight is reduced in winter in the northern hemisphere as the earth revolves in its orbit around the sun. With the sun lower on the horizon, we have weaker light and fewer daylight hours.[15]

What is the difference in sunlight intensity at different locations across the United States? I became a detective again. San Diego, Dr. Parry's PMS research site, is about 33° latitude north. Common sense suggests that there might be a higher number of light-affected women who live farther north where there is considerably less available sunlight. I wrote to NOAA, the National Oceanic and Atmospheric Administration, and asked for their weather records for San Diego, Denver, and Chicago.[16,17]

I found that Chicago receives 37-47 percent of the average possible sunshine for our latitude in the winter. Equally important, we spend most of our time indoors, away from the natural color balance of full spectrum light.

I thought I was not affected by light. But my curiosity pushed me to check it out. I purchased a professionally made light box. I was surprised and pleased to note that my efficiency increased. I found it easier to get papers off my desk and to return phone calls.

But why are some of us affected more severely in January, February, and March, when the days are getting longer? Scientists have discovered that the brain's pineal body acts like a built-in light meter.[18] It measures the intensity and color balance of light. The pineal also acts as a biological clock that times the length of the exposure. Our brains function like solar-powered batteries that run down when we don't get enough light. So even when we add additional sunlight, it takes time to recharge our batteries. Thus, light-affected people may feel worse in late winter although the days are lengthening.

I had another question. The news media in the U.S. is full of stories about depression around the December holidays. December 21 is our shortest day of the year. If light-related depression is common at that time in the northern hemisphere, does the increased light the southern hemisphere receives in December reduce such depression?

I wrote to an Australian Dalton Society colleague, Dr. Iain Esslemont. I asked him for his observations about depression during the December holidays, near their longest day of the year. Did psychologists and the media report an increase in depression?

Dr. Esslemont answered,

> In Australia, depression does not seem to be more marked during the holidays than at any other time, although an event for celebration is noted as a time for concern in someone who has suffered the loss of a loved one.[19]

Just as I suspected. Deceased or distant loved ones certainly are missed, but in Australia people do not go into severe depression in December as we often do in the northern hemisphere. That information plus studies and anecdotes in the United States indicate that light helps us cope with life's stresses.

Norman Rosenthal, M.D., included the following table in his enlightening book, *Seasons of the Mind*.[20] Although he was writing about SAD, I believe the same statistics (or higher) would apply to women with classic PMS and light sensitivity. Remember also that those of us who live farther north spend more time indoors.

Estimate of Percentage of Light-Affected People at Different Latitudes in the United States

Latitude	Regions	Severely affected(%)	Mild-Moderate(%)
45-50°	Washington state across the U.S. to northern Wisconsin, Michigan, and Maine	10.2	20.2
40-45°	Oregon across the U.S. to Chicago and New York	8.0	17.1
35-40°	Northern California across the U.S. to Missouri and Washington, D.C	5.8	13.9
30-35°	Southern California across the U.S. to Louisiana and South Carolina	3.6	10.6
25-30°	Mexico, southern Texas, and Florida	1.4	7.5

People in the far north are sharply affected by light changes throughout the year. The *Wall Street Journal Europe*[21] printed a front page article in February 1992 about using bright lights, or phototherapy, to "Help Swedes Lighten Up a Little." The article describes a hospital ward where depressed people arrive quietly at 6:00 AM and leave talking and laughing two hours later.

I was recently surprised and impressed to learn that it is illegal to use anything but full spectrum light in hospitals and medical facilities in Germany.[22]

I saw the light when it came to PMS and serotonin. Women with PMS need to lighten up!

Scientists have known for ages that light affects the reproductive cycle of animals. Some, such as cows and ewes, become fertile when light is reduced in the fall. This ensures that calves and lambs are born in the spring.[23]

In 1980 researchers became aware that light affects humans as well. In the far north, women may have very long cycles or almost cease menstruating entirely.[24,25] More human babies are born in the winter and spring, indicating more sexual interest and activity in the previous spring and summer.[26]

In 1967 researchers reported that sleeping under a 100 watt light bulb at midcycle (simulating the full moon) could regulate and stabilize women's cycles at 29 days, a lunar month.[27,28] In her book *Lunaception*, Louise Lacey states that 28 out of 30 women were able to stabilize their cycles in order to conceive or to avoid pregnancy.[29] Researchers confirmed this effect in 1991 using lower-wattage bulbs.[30] (I suggest you use a full spectrum bulb if you wish to try it. See the Resource Appendix.)

We do not yet know how much light each individual needs. However, we suspect that the amount of light the body needs generally increases with age. Could that be one of the reasons that PMS also generally increases with age? Could it be why retirees flock to the southern parts of the U.S.?

Henry Lahmeyer, M.D., director of the Department of Psychiatry at Northwestern University, works with SAD, Seasonal Affective Disorder. He noted, "Many [SAD] patients say they feel like they have a physical ailment, a flu that they just can't shake. They say they feel that they're in a fog. They notice they can't function at work. They're slow, they're not creative, and they just don't laugh anymore."[31]

I'm convinced. I see a definite correlation between light, PMS, and SAD.[32] In *Seasons of the Mind*, Norman Rosenthal, M.D., noted that four times as many women as men were affected by SAD.[33] That increase in light sensitivity may be partly related to the serotonin/melatonin drop during the last half of the cycle.

But another question arises—does it matter what kind of light we use?

One More Piece of the Puzzle

Light is important, but what kind? Research points to dramatic health benefits with full spectrum light. Full spectrum light has two parts: one visible, one invisible. The visible spectrum consists of all the colors of natural sunlight. Imagine a rainbow or light broken up by a prism.

John Ott, Sci.D. (Hon.), lighting pioneer, discovered that a balanced color range is essential to produce both male and female flowers.[34] While doing time-lapse photography under "cool white" fluorescent light, he noted that a pumpkin plant produced only male blossoms. Under "daylight white" fluorescent bulbs, the pumpkin produced only female blossoms. It required the full spectrum of light to produce both male and female blossoms.

Our eyes can only see a small portion of the electromagnetic spectrum, known as visible light. Our bodies, however, also respond to radiation just outside the range of visible light. Infrared light comes from near the red end of the spectrum. When it strikes our skin, we feel it as heat. Think of a red-hot electric burner or a heat lamp. Ultraviolet, or "black," light is near the opposite, violet end of the visible spectrum.

We derive health benefits from both ends of the spectrum, the *full* spectrum. Complete light energy from the sun is essential to life. We particularly need ultraviolet. If we get too much of it, we burn, but with too little, our bodies develop numerous health problems. Balance is the key.

Ultraviolet light is present all the time outdoors during the day, even on cloudy days. You may have heard that ultraviolet light is bad for us and that we must protect ourselves from it. That is partly correct and partly incorrect. Ultraviolet (UV) light is commonly divided into three sections depending on its wavelength: near-UV (UV-A), mid-UV (UV-B), and far-UV (UV-C).[35,36] UV-A tans us. UV-B stimulates the production of Vitamin D_3 in our skin[37] and is essential for the absorption of calcium into bones.[38] The natural skin oils produced after ultraviolet exposure are capable of killing bacteria.[39] Niels Finsen received the Nobel Prize in 1903 for successfully treating tuberculosis skin lesions with ultraviolet light. In fact, until penicillin was discovered in 1938, the preferred method of treating a wide variety of infectious diseases was exposure to the sun and its ultraviolet light, because sunlight was so effective in stimulating the patient's own immune system.

UV-C is another story. Although used in hospitals to kill bacteria and viruses, UV-C is widely considered to increase the risk of cancer. Fortunately, most of the UV-C that the sun gives off is blocked by the ozone layer of the earth's atmosphere. Still, it is clear that *over*exposure to the sun greatly increases your chance of developing skin cancer. Regular, moderate exposure, however, may actually decrease it. One rigorous study found that the incidence of malignant melanomas was considerably higher in office workers than in people who were regularly exposed to sunlight in their occupations or lifestyles. In fact, one of the lowest-risk groups was sunbathers. They were only half as likely to get malignant skin cancer as the office workers.[40]

In his book *Light: Medicine of the Future*,[41] Jacob Liberman, O.D., Ph.D., lists ten benefits of ultraviolet A and B. The following points are a synopsis of the research which he pulled together. For complete information, please get his book.

1. UV light activates the synthesis of vitamin D, which is a prerequisite for the absorption of calcium and other minerals from the diet.

    In a controlled study, the group receiving UV absorbed 40 percent more calcium from their diet than their counterparts who received no UV.[42,43,44,45,46,47]

2. UV light lowers blood pressure.

    One study reported that ultraviolet light dramatically lowered blood pressure after one treatment. The effect lasted five to six days.[48]

3. UV light increases the efficiency of the heart.

    In 18 of 20 people tested, cardiac output increased an average of 39 percent. In other words, their hearts became stronger and pumped more blood.[49]

4. UV light improves electrocardiogram (EKG) readings and blood profiles of individuals with atherosclerosis (hardening of the arteries).[50,51,52,53]

5. UV light reduces cholesterol.

    In one experiment, 97 percent of the patients had almost a 13 percent decrease in serum cholesterol levels two hours after their first exposure. Within this group, 86 percent maintained this level 24 hours later.[54]

6. UV light assists in weight loss.

    This may be because the UV stimulates the thyroid gland, which increases metabolism and thus burns calories.[55]

7. UV light is an effective treatment for psoriasis.

    The National Psoriasis Foundation reports that 80 percent of people suffering from this condition improve when exposed to UV.[56]

8. UV light is an effective treatment for many other diseases, including tuberculosis and asthma.[57,58,59]

9. UV light increases the level of sex hormones.

    One medical laboratory found that estrogen has a sharp peak of absorption in a portion of the UV-B range (290 nanometers). This finding indicates that estrogen is most efficient when a woman is exposed to UV wavelengths.[60]

10. UV light activates solitrol, an important hormone in the skin that works in conjunction with the pineal hormone melatonin.[61]

    Solitrol, possibly a form of vitamin D_3, influences the immune system as well as many of the body's regulatory centers.

As Dr. Liberman so thoroughly documents, ultraviolet light is beneficial.

To be most effective, light must be as close to sunlight proportions as possible, both in its visible color spectrum and in ultraviolet A and B. Unfortunately, our regular indoor lighting is weakest at the blue end of the spectrum (where natural sunlight is strongest) and has very little or no ultraviolet. Incandescent (screw-in) bulbs emit too much orange and red; cool white fluorescent tubes put out too much green and yellow. We do get color-balanced light through clear plastic and glass windows, but windows still block ultraviolet. Tinted car windows block the ultraviolet and change the color balance. Most contact lenses also block UV, and colored ones change the color balance. Our bodies are too often deprived of adequate color and of ultraviolet.

The connection with contacts surprised me. I told a Chicago woman with PMS of the importance of balanced, full spectrum light. When she stopped wearing her blue contacts, her PMS disappeared! Without her colored lenses, the full spectrum of visible and ultraviolet light entered her eyes. (For information on where to get ultraviolet transmitting glasses and contacts, check the Resource Appendix.)

It's time we paid attention to the light around us. It is important to have full spectrum (full color with UV) light in our lives.

Here are some suggestions you can begin today:

1. Walk outside at lunch time or anytime during the day. There is more light outside, even on a cloudy day, than in the best-lit office or home.

2. Leave your glasses, contacts, or sunglasses off as much as possible—or get full spectrum UV-transmitting lenses.

3. Move your desk or couch closer to the window so that you get the best color-balanced light possible.

4. Correct the light around you.

   a. Change your incandescent bulbs to full spectrum incandescents or, better yet, full spectrum Capsulites. (These are fluorescent bulbs designed to fit in an incandescent fixture.)

b. Switch your cool white fluorescent tubes to full spectrum fluorescents.

c. Check with your health care practitioner about buying a *full spectrum* light box. If your doctor prescribes it for you, it may be covered by insurance. You'll find a sample insurance claim letter with the Resource Appendix for your doctor to use. See the Resource Appendix for lighting sources.

5. Work during the daytime if possible. Night shifts or swing shifts can upset sleep cycles. (Classic PMS is a sleep disorder.) Whatever your work requires, try to stick close to the same sleep schedule even on the weekend.

6. Take a walk in the morning. Get out in that early morning light. 95 percent of people with light-related symptoms find that morning light is best for them. Most of us have an internal 25-hour clock. When you are exposed to early morning light, you reset that clock to match our planet's 24-hour clock.

Light affects us when it enters the eyes and when it strikes the skin. Most of the beneficial brain-chemistry effects are produced by light entering the eyes. This does not mean that we must look at the sun or at a full spectrum bulb. Ultraviolet will reflect off of our surroundings just as visible light does. Remember the positive physiological effects of ultraviolet light striking the skin, such as lower cholesterol and stronger bones.

Incidentally, beware of tanning beds. The high concentration of UV-A light they put out is quite different from the proportions of UV-A and UV-B in natural sunlight. Tanning with an unnaturally high proportion of UV-A light is dangerous.

Does light need to be extremely bright to affect us? No. One study of SAD people documented a three-fold improvement in mood with a not-very-bright 2500 lux full spectrum light.[62]

Women with classic PMS may have relatives with a history of migraines, sleep disorders, or alcohol abuse. If you have low levels of serotonin and melatonin, you may have PMS symptoms during the day and not sleep well at night. You may get up during the night to go to the bathroom, you may wake up just to turn over, or you may sleep very deeply for long hours and still wake up tired. Both extremes are indications of poor sleep patterns, frequently caused by low levels of melatonin.

Researchers are investigating a possible link between postpartum depression and light.[41] Other studies are underway that investigate the effect of light on menstrual cycle length, on fertility, and on shift work. Keep your eyes open for new research.

With additional light, especially full spectrum light, many women with PMS (and their families!) feel better. So—

LIGHTEN UP!

My search was over.

But wait a minute. Some women *still* had symptoms. What else was going on?

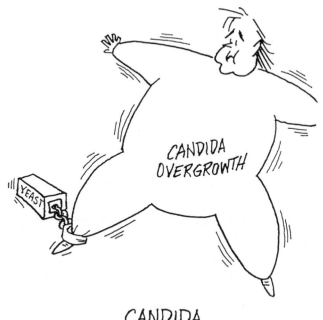

CANDIDA
— OR WHY DO I STILL
FEEL SO BAD?

The laboratory tests say you're okay. Then why do you feel so bad? The culprit could be a fairly new diagnosis, one that was only identified in the 1980s: Candida albicans.

After listening for several years to women with PMS, I recognized that Candida is another hidden cause of PMS. Candida is a one-celled yeast organism which, along with good organisms, lives in everyone's bodies. Usually our immune system keeps their numbers under control, but sometimes Candida grows out of control and produces symptoms. As a disease, it often appears first as thrush or a vaginal infection. Anyone, man, woman, or child, who has an overgrowth of Candida and the resulting imbalance of bad to good organisms will have lots of miserable symptoms.

People at risk for Candida overgrowth have a history of:

- Antibiotics
- Birth control pills
- Pregnancies
- Steroids—Prednisone and cortisone
- High stress
- High sugar intake
- Poor diet

Over time these people develop a weakened immune system which can no longer keep the Candida under control.

Because Candida causes so many symptoms common to other conditions, the medical community has difficulty recognizing it. It is also controversial because no routine lab test yet exists which measures the amount of live Candida in the body. Since Candida shows up in nearly every blood test and stool culture, it is frequently ignored when it comes to evaluating how much is there. Only a few laboratories in the U.S. specialize in quantifying Candida levels, and these laboratories are rarely used. Instead, symptoms and medical and genetic histories are used to provide *The Missing Diagnosis*, as Orian Truss, M.D., called it in the first book about Candida in 1983.[1]

Like PMS, Candida affects different body systems to different extents. Candida overcolonization occurs in mucosal areas, such as the intestines, vagina, and sinuses. Like weeds growing in a garden, these yeast colonies grow rapidly and cause tissue damage where they grow.

Each Candida cell also releases toxins when it dies. These poisons travel throughout the body and can cause symptoms in the nervous, skeletal, muscular, respiratory, dermatologic (skin), endocrine, and immune systems—symptoms such as depression, fatigue, asthma, coughing, itching, hives, rashes, and head and body aches.

These variations are clearly described in one of the early books about Candida, *The Yeast Connection,* by William Crook,

M.D., which was published in 1984.[2] (His most recent book, published in 1995, is *The Yeast Connection and the Woman.*) I must admit that when I first read Dr. Crook's book, I threw it away. It seemed to suggest that Candida caused everything except flat feet and hangnails! Thanks to some women who thought I could be educated, I took another look at Candida. I owe an apology to Dr. Crook. He was right.

A Short Essay on
Yeast Infections,
Candida,
Candida Albicans,
or Atypical Candidiasis.
(Hint: They're all the same thing.)

Candida albicans, a yeast organism, can be detected in nearly every one of us by the time we are six months old. However, when the overgrowth first appears, it's generally a minor infection of the vagina or the mouth and known as a yeast infection or as thrush. It also frequently appears as diarrhea.

In a healthy individual, a strong immune system and an abundance of good microorganisms keep Candida under control. The yeast organism competes with the good bacteria in the intestinal, respiratory, and reproductive tract. However, Candida multiplies rapidly when our systems get out of balance.

But why would a vaginal infection (or a Candida infection elsewhere in the body) cause mental and emotional disruptions? That didn't make sense to me.

Laboratory research shows that the Candida organism releases 79 different toxins into the body as it dies.[3] These toxins enter the blood stream and travel throughout the body. Large colonies of these yeast organisms can cause confusion, fatigue, irritability, and severe depression, as well as physical symptoms such as migraines, muscle and joint aches, and intestinal upsets. Because Candida damages the intestinal wall, Candida toxins and large food molecules can go through the intestinal wall, a condition known as "leaky gut". Our immune system identifies these large, partially digested food particles as invaders, provoking an allergic response. (We'll get to that section later.)

One of the toxins, acetaldehyde, makes red blood cells abnormally rigid. This impairs circulation and reduces oxygen delivery to each cell in the body. Acetaldehyde also inhibits acetylcholine, a neurotransmitter in the brain. Low levels of acetylcholine can lead to erratic thinking, poor short-term memory, and deranged behavior. Does this sound familiar?

No parent is surprised when a sick child is cranky because they know that physical symptoms often have emotional components. When people have a headache or the flu, their energy level and outlook is down. People with Candida typically have similar, but often more severe, symptoms. The *Journal of the American Medical Association* notes that depression, a frequent Candida symptom, improves as Candida is brought under control.[4]

Candida usually sets up large colonies in the intestinal system. It can cause bloating, gas, heartburn, diarrhea, and constipation. Because Candida needs sugar to live, it is frequently mistaken for hypoglycemia, or low blood sugar. People with Candida may experience fatigue and mental fog or become emotional between meals, but a glucose tolerance test doesn't indicate hypoglycemia. They may even feel better briefly when they eat something sweet because sugar feeds Candida, temporarily reducing the flow of toxins from dying yeast cells. The symptoms reappear when some of the organisms complete their short life cycles and die. (In fact, diabetics and others with high blood sugar levels commonly do have a Candida overgrowth because their high blood sugar levels constantly feed the Candida.)

Candida can cause vaginitis, cystitis, and menstrual irregularities. It is even implicated in some cases of endometriosis and infertility. In the respiratory system, Candida can cause earaches, sinus problems, nasal drainage, sore throats, bronchitis, or coughing. It frequently causes headaches and fatigue. Some people with Candida experience adult onset acne. Others develop hives or severe chemical sensitivities. Some people suffer from symptoms in many areas, while others find that they have one area that is severely affected.

Candida overgrowth can be caused by several factors. Broad spectrum antibiotics, such as tetracycline, are particularly harmful because they destroy the good Candida-controlling bacteria along with the targeted pathogens. Steroids, such as cortisone and Prednisone, suppress the immune system's ability to control yeast growth. People may take antibiotics or steroids over the course of many years with only a gradual deterioration of health. Then, seemingly all of a sudden, their immune systems can no longer cope with the overgrowth of Candida. When this happens, Candida, a yeast organism which grows more rapidly than the good, health-supporting microorganisms, has additional space in which to multiply. The result is an imbalance of microorganisms, causing people to feel ill. Think of it like a lawn—as long as the grass is healthy, few weeds appear, but if the grass gets thin, weeds sprout quickly.

Though it occurs in men, women, and children, women are especially prone to Candida. Women take antibiotics more often for urinary tract infections and for acne. Also, the female hormone progesterone stimulates Candida growth.[5] Progesterone levels increase during the last half of the menstrual cycle, during pregnancy, and when taking birth control pills and hormone supplements such as Provera. As a result, Candida symptoms in women frequently increase before the menstrual period. Symptoms which were previously mild or unnoticed can become debilitating and severe. The increased numbers of Candida organisms release more toxins into our bodies as they complete their short life cycles and die. Since the Candida die-off occurs before a woman's period when her progesterone levels are dropping, and because Candida and classic PMS have similar symptoms, *atypical Candidiasis is often mistaken for PMS.* To complicate matters, many women have both conditions at the same time. Some women get their PMS under control only to find that they feel terrible again before their periods a few years later, not because their PMS has come back, but because they have a Candida overgrowth.

The yeast can also interfere with our hormone signals by creating molecules that look like our own natural hormones.[6] Perhaps the presence of Candida albicans is why research has shown that PMS-like symptoms can be present regardless of the level of progesterone in the body or the ratio of progesterone to estrogen.

I was surprised to learn that women can have severe atypical Candida (or Candidiasis) without having a vaginal infection. But since men also can have Candidiasis, people obviously do not have to have a vaginal yeast infection to have a Candida overgrowth. Candida can live in all mucosal areas (intestine, vagina, sinus, etc.), but the overgrowth may cause problems in only one area.

Some family members and health professionals do not see the relationship to the menstrual cycle since Candida is present all month. They may say that the symptoms are "all in our heads" and suggest counseling. While women experiencing the chaos of PMS may benefit from the emotional support of counseling, the cause of the symptoms is physical, not psychological. If your PMS doesn't clear up completely within two to three days of starting your period, or if your PMS symptoms go away, only to return around days four to six of your flow, look into Candida. (See pattern five in Chapter Three.)

In addition to a history of antibiotics, birth control pills, and pregnancies, greater sugar consumption during the last half of your cycle is an additional clue that you could have a Candida problem. The yeast needs sugar (or bread, pasta, or alcohol) to provide food for its reproduction. Unfortunately, these high sugar levels coupled with higher progesterone levels during the last two weeks of the cycle accelerate the Candida growth.

Now for the good news: *Candida albicans can be controlled.* It can be completely reversed. If this is the cause of your PMS, you can return to full health—with a little work. A four-pronged approach is recommended:

- Build up overall health
- Reduce Candida overgrowth

- Restrict foods which feed Candida
- Eliminate mold from your environment

Build up overall body health

Two main products, vitamins and acidophilus, help build up the body's systems. A high quality, yeast-free multivitamin-mineral helps to strengthen the immune system so it can fight the Candida. If you can't locate one in your area, check the Resource Appendix for sources.

Acidophilus is one of the good microorganisms which needs to be present in the body. Since it is used to make yogurt, eating yogurt increases the amount of acidophilus in the body. You may have heard about curing mild vaginal infections by eating yogurt. It does help. However, when you eat yogurt, be sure it is plain yogurt with a live acidophilus culture. Skip the ones with sugar, fruit, or aspartame (NutraSweet or Equal). Sugar and fruit feed the Candida; aspartame interferes with the serotonin levels involved in classic PMS. You can cook with plain yogurt or add cinnamon and nuts to it. (When you feel better, you can add fresh fruit.) Higher levels of acidophilus, available in pill or powder form, are even better at reimplanting the good microorganisms in the intestines and displacing Candida. Read the label and choose one that supplies *billions* of *live* acidophilus microorganisms. Again, if you can't find a quality source, check the Resource Appendix.

Incidentally, if you suspect that you had high levels of Candida before giving birth, or if your PMS started after a pregnancy, please take a look at your child's health. The baby may have been infected at birth. If he or she had intestinal upsets, colic, thrush, frequent diaper rashes, sleeping difficulties, colds, or ear infections, Candida overgrowth is a likely culprit (as are food allergies). A healthy intestinal balance is easily established at that age by giving the child children's sugarless vitamins and bifida supplements. Bifida is a beneficial microorganism, like acidophilus, that displaces Candida in the intestinal tract. It is used until the child is six.

Reduce Candida overgrowth

While you are building up the general health of your body by taking acidophilus and vitamins, you can speed your recovery by taking caprylic acid and garlic to reduce the Candida overgrowth. Our bodies make small amounts of caprylic acid (among other things) from fats and oils, such as olive oil, corn oil, and butter, but the amount produced by the body is insufficient to reverse atypical Candidiasis. Caprylic acid has antifungal properties and has very little, if any, negative effect on normal intestinal bacteria.[7] Caprylic acid dissolves the cell wall of the Candida, killing the yeast cell and releasing its toxins into the body, where they cause symptoms until they are excreted.[8] Some doctors prescribe Nystatin, which also kills Candida.[9] Other health care providers recommend a grapefruit seed extract.

Garlic is another weapon in the fight against Candida. Garlic kills twenty different kinds of fungus, including Candida albicans.[10] Recent scientific research clearly indicates that it has many health benefits in addition to its effectiveness against Candida. Garlic is effective against viruses. Studies also show that it helps to lower cholesterol.[11] Other studies show that it is a powerful antioxidant. I still take it, even though I no longer have a Candida overgrowth.

You can buy "odorless" garlic pills so you won't drive your friends away. I prefer brands that contain the whole garlic clove. Be sure to read the label. If you don't take the whole garlic, you may not get the compounds that are most effective.

If Candida has invaded the urinary tract, cranberry extract (without sugar or NutraSweet) and cranberry pills are effective,[12] especially when taken with garlic.

Many sufferers of Candidiasis experience a die-off response shortly after beginning their Candida control program as the Candida organisms die and release toxins into the bloodstream. This die-off may reveal itself as fatigue, headaches, sinus drainage, or digestive or emotional upsets. Many people say it feels like having the flu. These symptoms are temporary, usually lasting only for the first week or so of therapy. Many people begin to notice improvement in a few days. The sometimes uncomfortable die-off period is well worth going through. Several grams of vitamin C daily will reduce the die-off effect. Your health care professional may recommend that you start taking caprylic acid at low levels and gradually raise it as the Candida concentration decreases and you begin to feel better. This will help reduce the die-off effect.

Restrict foods which feed Candida

Taking pills is easy for most of us. You'll be happy to know that you won't have to take them forever. The hard part may be restricting the foods which feed Candida. And it is essential not to eat things that nourish Candida. Feeding the Candida while you kill it off only produces more dying Candida, more toxins, and more nasty symptoms. Your recovery will be much faster if you don't nourish the Candida while you are taking supplements to reduce it.

I have found that the most important dietary restriction is to temporarily eliminate sugar and fermented and aged foods. Sugar, of course, encourages the growth of Candida. Restricting sugar in your diet means restricting sugar in all forms, including fruit and fruit juice (temporarily). During the recovery period, you must eliminate fermented foods, such as alcohol, soy sauce, vinegar, salad dressings, catsup, and mustards (which contain vinegar), because they are made with or contain yeast. Aged foods, such as cheese, and mushrooms (an edible fungi) must also be excluded. It is also important to avoid foods containing yeast, such as bread, cake, doughnuts, and pizza. All of these foods should be avoided until you feel better; they can then be added back into your diet. A yeast-free vitamin and mineral supplement is also important.

These food restrictions are temporary. When you feel better again, reintroduce each food from the problem food list one at a time and find out if it still bothers you. Most will probably be fine. If you have a reaction, you can decide what to do. If you want to feel bad, eat it; if you want to feel good, avoid it.

Think of the symptoms you get when you have a cold or an allergic reaction. They are caused by your immune system reacting to an invader. These symptoms, plus the toxic reaction caused by the dying yeast's toxins, can be quite annoying and can make us feel miserable during the early stages of our counterattack on Candida. Our immune system recognizes yeast and yeast products (like vinegar and alcohol) as part of the Candida infection it is fighting, and it responds by attacking the invader—causing more symptoms.

So what can you eat? Lots! Eating a variety of foods is a good idea. Think of this as a chance to experiment with new foods, a chance to make new friends. You can try new chicken and fish recipes. Breads made with baking soda instead of yeast, such as Irish soda bread and sugar-free corn bread, are excellent choices. Many people make tortilla sandwiches. Lemon and olive oil salad dressings are great substitutes for vinegar and oil dressings.

Many people feel better when they cut back on preservatives in their diet. Frozen vegetables are healthier than canned ones. Think "rainbow diet." Variety and color are important. Fresh, not old or moldy, vegetables are especially good. Also, drinking lots of water flushes toxins from the body.

Incidentally, many people sometimes have a toxic reaction to peanuts, peanut butter, and pistachios. This isn't a Candida overgrowth or food sensitivity reaction. A mold that often grows on these nuts produces aflatoxin, a powerful poison, and will make anyone sick.

One study printed in the *Journal of the American Medical Association* in the fall of 1992 tested the prescription drug Nystatin, which is similar to caprylic acid, against Candida.[13] Some people got better; some did not. However, the participants were not asked to follow a restricted diet, nor were they asked about acidophilus, vitamins, and minerals. Some probably took supplements on their own; others doubtless did not. An antifungal alone is not enough. Let me emphasize this: an antifungal alone is not enough.[14] You must restrict Candida-feeding foods temporarily.

Eliminate mold

Eliminate as much mold from your home and office environments as possible. Environmental mold, mildew, and fungi, which often grow in bathrooms, basements, and closets, must be reduced. Chlorine bleach, Lysol, and Melaleuca (Tea Tree Oil) are effective antibacterial/antifungals. Cleaning may need to be repeated frequently during a wet season. An effective way to slow the growth of environmental molds is to place open containers of baking soda throughout the house. If you use chemicals, be sure to use them with the windows open and keep them away from small children.

Although women with a Candida overgrowth will feel better even during the first month on this program, most people need to stay on the program for three to four months to start feeling "normal" again. However, even when a positive response occurs rapidly, many people find that they need six to ten months to really control their Candida. It often takes several months for the good microorganisms to reestablish themselves after the Candida population is reduced.

If someone stops the program too early, Candida may come back. I have found that a woman needs to have two symptom-free cycles before her pill intake can be lowered and her diet broadened. If she stops the program too soon, she will have to start over again before the year is out.

After two symptom-free cycles, a woman's immune system is strong enough to keep her Candida under control despite the Candida-stimulating progesterone levels that come at the end of her cycle. At that point she can gradually expand her diet and begin to eliminate acidophilus and caprylic acid. She should continue to take vitamins and minerals, possibly garlic, and keep eating well. If she does not feel well after several cycles on an anti-Candida program, it's time to look for parasites or food allergies. Keep reading—we'll cover them.

In the interest of general health, I strongly encourage every woman to follow an anti-Candida regimen for a few months before a pregnancy to reduce the risk of Candida-caused postpartum depression. Some women who thought that they were infertile have been able to become pregnant after reducing their Candida overgrowth.

What fun to listen to these women as they begin to feel better:

"This is fascinating! I can see a definite cause and effect relationship between taking the pills [acidophilus, vitamins, garlic, and caprylic acid] and the release of symptoms. "—from a physics professor.

"I'm feeling better, but I'm almost afraid to talk about it! Maybe it will go away. "—from a registered nurse.

"I'm not crying anymore! And I used to be a puddle all the time. "—from a writer/producer in public relations.

"I used to be so embarrassed because of gas. Do you know how great it is not to have to avoid people?!"—from an office worker.

"I can breathe again!"—from a woman with recurring sinus infections.

"I can't believe that I don't have to go to the emergency ward for a narcotic shot for my premenstrual migraines any longer. "—from a businesswoman.

"I felt like a teenager again with my adult-onset acne. Now that's gone and I understand that it was my body trying to excrete excess Candida toxins. "—from a 36-year-old.

"I have energy I haven't felt for years!"—from a woman who works out regularly.

"I've had severe headaches since my ten-year-old was born. No one could find the cause. And now they're gone!"—from a teacher.

"For the past thirteen years I had diarrhea for ten days before my period and the first three days of my flow. I couldn't leave the house, so I ran a home day care business. Now I can go anywhere and not ask where the bathroom is as soon as I enter the store!! "—from a thrilled mom.

"The vaginal and bladder infections I've had for years have stopped."—from several women.

"I can hardly believe it. In addition to feeling well, I'm back to my early 20s weight with no effort."—from several who had tried various diet plans.

Candida is something which we *all* must rule in or rule out. The history and symptom questionnaire which follows is quite accurate. Even if you don't have vaginal infections and are skeptical, fill it out! Candida may be part of your PMS puzzle, too.

It is impossible to do justice to the complexity of Candida in one chapter. It has been called a twentieth century epidemic. If you suspect you might have a problem, check the Select Bibliography for more information.[15,16,17,18,19,20,21,22] I particularly recommend the Crook books for their numerous examples and the Trowbridge book for its strong medical foundation.[23,24]

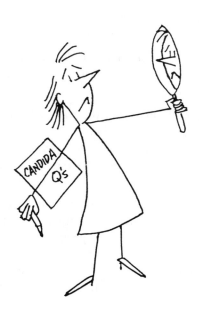

CANDIDA QUESTIONNAIRE

Answer each question "yes" or "no" by circling the appropriate word.

PART I. MEDICAL HISTORY

A. Have you had (or do you now have)
1. Thyroid treatments
    (or thyroid tests with borderline results?)   yes no
2. Diabetes?   yes no
3. Cancer in any form?   yes no
4. Hypoglycemia?   yes no

B. Have you had
1. Operation(s)?   yes no
2. Catheterization(s)?   yes no
3. Anti-cancer medication(s)?   yes no
4. Radiation treatment(s)?   yes no

C. Have you taken
1.   Antibiotics?   yes no
2.   Tetracycline or Erythromycin for acne?   yes no
3.   Oral contraceptives (women only)?   yes no
4.   Progesterone (women only)?   yes no
5.   Fertility drugs (women only)?   yes no
6.   Oral or injected cortisone (includes Prednisone)   yes no

D. Do you live (or have you lived) in a
1.   Damp climate?   yes no
2.   Moldy house?   yes no
3.   Area of foggy beaches?   yes no

E. Do you have (or have you ever had)
1.   An alcohol problem?   yes no

F. Do you use (or have you ever used)
1.   Marijuana?   yes no
2.   Cocaine?   yes no
3.   Heroin?   yes no

G. Have you had recurrent viral or bacterial infections?   yes no

H. Have you had recurrent yeast infections at any time?
1.   Vaginal (women only)   yes no
2.   Nail   yes no
3.   Thrush   yes no
4.   Jock itch (men only)   yes no

PART II. PRESENT SITUATION

A. Are your symptoms worse
1.   When raking dry leaves?   yes no
2.   In a damp basement or office?   yes no
3.   On rainy or humid days?   yes no

B. Do you crave
1.   Sugar?   yes no
2.   Breads?   yes no
3.   Milk products?   yes no
4.   Alcohol?   yes no

C. Are you uncomfortable when in contact with
1.   Smoke (any type)?   yes no

2. Fumes (any type)?   yes no
3. Agricultural chemicals?   yes no
4. Perfume, cologne, soaps, laundry detergent?   yes no

PART III. DIGESTIVE SYSTEM SYMPTOMS

Are the following symptoms present?
1. Gas/abdominal distention   yes no
2. Diarrhea or constipation   yes no
3. Hemorrhoids   yes no
4. Anal itching   yes no
5. Mucus in stools   yes no
6. Heartburn/indigestion   yes no
7. Bad breath   yes no
8. Constant hunger   yes no
9. Food allergies   yes no
10. Weight gain or loss without change in diet   yes no
11. Thick white or yellow coating on tongue in morning yes no

PART IV. MENTAL/HEAD SYMPTOMS

Are the following symptoms present?
1. Difficulty in concentration   yes no
2. Short attention span   yes no
3. Memory retention difficulty   yes no
4. Fogginess, spaciness   yes no
5. Excessive sleepiness   yes no
6. Headaches   yes no
7. Depression and/or suicidal thoughts   yes no
8. Mood swing   yes no
9. Irritability/anger   yes no
10. Mental confusion   yes no

PART V. HORMONAL SYMPTOMS

Are the following symptoms present?
1. Premenstrual syndrome (women only)   yes no
2. Yeast infection week before period (women only) yes no
3. Endometriosis (women only)   yes no
4. Menstrual irregularities (women only)   yes no

5.	Decreased sexual desire	yes no
6.	Yeast infection or jock itch after intercourse	yes no
7.	Infertility without identifiable cause	yes no
8.	Impotence (men only)	yes no

PART VI. MISCELLANEOUS SYMPTOMS

Are the following symptoms present?

1.	Tightness in chest	yes no
2.	Heart palpitations	yes no
3.	Urinary frequency, urgency, burning	yes no
4.	Postnasal drip	yes no
5.	Muscle or joint pains	yes no
6.	Cold hands or feet	yes no
7.	Poor coordination, balance problems	yes no
8.	Water retention (edema)	yes no
9.	Swallowing difficulties/sore throats	yes no
10.	Sinus headaches/earaches	yes no
11.	Eyes burning, tearing	yes no
12.	Itching, scaling skin	yes no
13.	Prostatitis (men only)	yes no

Total possible "yes" answers for women is 75; for men 69. A score higher than 50 means you are very likely to have an atypical Candida infection. 40 or more indicates Candida probably is affecting your health. With a score of 30 or more, a Candida illness may be present.[1] I have also met women with very low scores who felt much better after following a Candida reduction program. Thanks to Vicki Glassburn for permission to use the above questionnaire, first used in her book, *Who Killed Candida?*

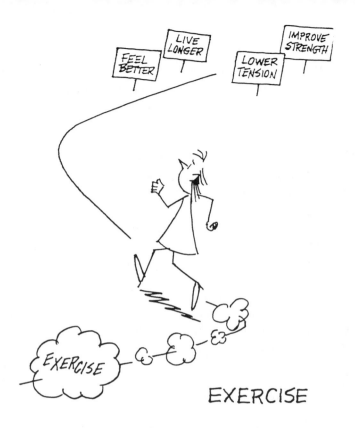

FEEL BETTER

LIVE LONGER

LOWER TENSION

IMPROVE STRENGTH

EXERCISE

EXERCISE

You may have been wondering when I would mention exercise. You're right. It is a very important piece of our PMS puzzle.

We can all recite numerous reasons to exercise: it's good for our cardiovascular systems, it improves strength and stamina, removes toxins, and increases endorphins—the feel-good hormones. Exercise lowers anxiety and tension by lowering adrenalin levels. It has also been shown to ward off cancer and increase longevity. And, of course, exercise contributes to weight control.

I listed weight control last because our society places too much emphasis on being thin. One woman who has a good perspective on exercise commented, "Exercise brings me positive energy, optimism, and joy. Exercise is not about being a size eight. It's about feeling better, relieving my stress, and helping me cope with life."

There were days when I ached so badly and was so tired that I could hardly get out of bed. Fortunately for me, my neighbor was an aerobics instructor and held classes in her home. It was so close, and the class really cared whether I was there or not, so I went. Sometimes it was easier to go than to explain why I didn't make it! Much to my surprise, no matter how hard it was to get there, I always felt better after class.

I recently read three studies which found that aerobic exercise causes both physical and emotional PMS symptoms to decline, while weight training causes physical symptoms alone to decline. Those who did not increase their exercise continued to have their usual level of symptoms.[1,2] The aerobic training group also did significantly better in stressful situations.[3]

Research indicates that those of us who are the most sedentary reap the most benefit when we start moving. Start today! Even two minutes is more than none. There were days when I didn't think I could do even two minutes. But when I got myself moving, I found I could continue. Besides the immediate emotional lift, a ten-minute walk gives a full hour of increased energy.

You'll feel better today *and* live a longer and healthier life. My personal goal is to stay healthy until I die. I'm not a fitness fanatic, yet I enjoy working outside, walking, cycling, dancing, and water and snow skiing. You may prefer swimming, tennis, or something else—or a mix of activities. Choose activities you enjoy, because those are the ones you will stay with. A brisk thirty-minute walk three or four times a week is great.

Design your exercise program to suit yourself. There are many ways to exercise. I needed a friend or class to encourage me. Other people prefer to exercise alone and use that time for meditation. You will find it easier to exercise when you follow your natural inclination, whether for solitary, quiet exercise, or for the social experience of a class.

You choose the type of exercise and the time to do it. You choose whether to be with a partner or alone. And as the seasons or your interests change, you can change what you do. You might decide to play racquetball, tennis, basketball, or volleyball, or go horseback riding.

Keep in mind that the purpose is to be active and have fun. It's not necessary to win all the time when you *play* competitive games. Exercise can be fun even when you're not highly skilled.

Exercise specialists tell us that the fastest way to get into shape is to do interval training.[4] Interval training occurs when you repeatedly push your body and then back off.

Exercise intensity is measured by how hard our heart is working. When we exercise, our bodies become more efficient and can do the same work with less effort. This training effect explains why people who exercise feel younger and more vigorous and alert. With regular exercise, everyday tasks become easier and require less effort, because exercise makes our bodies—and our brains—more capable and efficient. People who regularly exercise have a biological age which is younger than their chronological age.[5] They handle stress better and get sick less often. They even report feeling happier.

In fact, scientists say that the older a person is, the more he or she will benefit from exercising. Moderate exercise might add 20 percent to a young person's strength and endurance, but the same level of exercise, scaled to match an older person's capability, can nearly *double* an 80-year-old's strength and endurance!

We have been taught that we can determine how hard we are exercising by taking our heart rate as a percentage of our maximum safe heart rate. Thus someone who is running fairly fast might reach 80 percent of her maximum rate, while a slow walk might only get her heart pumping at 50 percent of its maximum. The following chart shows how different heart rates, from 50-90 percent of maximum, translate into those target ranges. Since hearts come in different sizes, however, some exercise physiologists are now suggesting that a better gauge of exertion is our sense of what each level feels like.[6] Small hearts will pump faster to move the same amount of blood as a larger heart.

Today's guideline: if you can carry on a conversation while you exercise without gasping for breath, you're probably in a good range for you to burn fat. If you want to build aerobic capacity, endurance, and muscle tone, you need to work harder. Your aerobic threshold and perceived exertion level will change from day to day. Listen to your own body, not an arbitrary rule.

		Age			
		30	40	50	
	50%	95	90	85	Very light
Percent of	60%	114	108	102	Fairly light
maximum	70%	133	126	119	Moderate
heart rate	80%	152	144	136	Hard
	85%	162	153	145	Hard
	90%	171	162	153	Very hard

Perceived exertion (right side)

Probable heart rate
(depends on size of heart
as well as condition)

If you haven't exercised in a while you might be surprised at how little it takes to get your heart pumping, but remember, you are going to improve, and feel better, much faster than someone who exercises already. If you have not been exercising for a while, please check with your doctor before you start.

Did you know that you can increase the value of your exercise by thinking of positive images while you're exercising? If you can't go outside, imagine yourself in the warm, healing sun with a gentle breeze blowing while you work out. Challenge your imagination to create something positive for yourself.

There is a cumulative effect to exercise. Ten minutes of walking the dog, ten minutes of dancing, and ten minutes of stretching while you put the dishes away add up to thirty minutes a day.

These suggestions can help you increase your daily activity:

- Walk to the store instead of driving, or park at the far end of the parking lot. If you ride public transportation, get off a stop or two before your destination and walk.

- Take the stairs instead of the elevator. Walk those reports to the office on another floor or in the next building.

- Pedal your exercise bike while watching TV, reading, or watching the kids.

- Play tag with the kids—or play catch, or baseball, or swim, bicycle, hike, or roller skate.

- Take a walk during your lunch hour—outside whenever possible.

It's never too late to start exercising. My Aunt Mary had a heart attack at 70. Her doctor recommended that she walk a mile a day. She decided to walk in a different direction each day of the week and watch the changes that happened in the world around her. She observed plants, and birds, and animals, and children, and building construction, and light, and changes in the weather. Her husband gave her an aluminum-framed backpack when she was 75. She loved it and went on longer hikes and overnight camping trips. She eventually wrote a book, *Seven Half-Miles from Home*.[7] Even though she died in her mid-80s, I can still hear her say, "Anyone can walk a half-mile away from home and then come back—*in any weather*." Aunt Mary is an inspiration to me. Even though she had a serious health problem, she found a way to get up and start exercising.

It is important that you make the changes for *yourself*—not for anyone else. *You* are the one who will feel better.

One last point: remember the additional benefits of full spectrum light—lower cholesterol, stronger bones, better infection resistance?[8] See you outside!

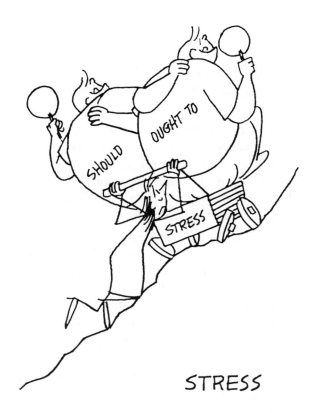

STRESS

Stress. We all have it. It does not *cause* PMS but can make the symptoms worse. The question is how can we deal with or reduce the stress we have.

We view some stresses as good, such as a new house, job, or baby. Other stresses we consider bad, such as too many demands on our time or finances. Both good and bad stresses can cause worry, fear, or anxiety. The mind/body system doesn't know the difference; it only perceives too many changes or demands. We may become short-tempered or depressed, or we may develop physical symptoms. We feel frustrated because we seem to be unable to control our lives. Often we are even more upset by the emotions that too much stress causes. We may feel guilty about our behavior but not know how to change it. Because both good and bad stresses ask our bodies to respond, we need to know how to manage these demands and reduce their effects.

High stress reveals a lack of balance in our lives. The first key is to recognize that we're out of balance. It may take time to correct the imbalances in our bodies and in our schedules, but it can be done.

Ask yourself if you are doing what you want to do. Also ask what is *really* expected of you. When I was trying to reduce my perfectionist tendencies, I found it helpful to tease myself. When I got uptight about my dirty kitchen floor, I would tell myself that if a dirt floor was good enough for Grandma, a pioneer woman who lived in a sod house, it was good enough for me.

If friends or family were coming to visit, I reminded myself that they were coming to see *me*, not to inspect my housekeeping. I remember the time when I had a 15-month-old, a new baby, and a new house. When people came over to see us, I thought I had to have the closets clean and the dirty clothes baskets empty! That doesn't happen any more. I now invite women who have an orderliness attack before their period to come over and clean my house.

Even though a *lot* of clutter bothers me, I also believe that seeing things scattered about—toys, books, magazines, hobbies—is a sign of a house filled with activities and interests. As long as the piles move occasionally because someone is interested in them, they don't bother me.

One of my friends taught me to clean house *after* children's birthday parties. That made a lot of sense. The house would definitely need cleaning then and the children didn't care if there was a little dust around.

What are your "ought tos" or "shoulds?" Ask yourself if they are really necessary. A bumper sticker I got for an over-committed friend reads, "Of course I *can* do it; the question is, do I *want* to?"

Also ask yourself, do you *really* have time? Or are you actually avoiding something else, such as an unpleasant home or work situation?

Is your "to do" list too long? Perhaps the responsibility of household tasks could be spread among family members. Even little ones can learn to fold laundry and set the table. (Teach them during the good part of your cycle when you have more patience.) Ask older family members to contribute at least two hours a week to the general welfare.

On a day when you are feeling good, make a list of the things you need to do. Then look at it again. Cross off the things that are not essential. You don't need the extra guilt of an unfinished list!

Next, prioritize your list. Then tackle the most important jobs first. Every major project can be broken down into smaller parts. You'll probably feel more productive at the end of the day if you spend time on your most important projects and let the little ones slide.

Even when I'm healthy and I have my tasks prioritized, there are days when I don't finish my list. Could it be that I'm overscheduled? (The answer is frequently yes, but I'm learning.) You may have the same pattern. Try to be understanding of yourself, and do keep in mind that a day has only twenty-four hours!

Start Your Own Peace Plan

Do you remember the Golden Rule? "Do unto others as you would have them do unto you." I'd like to change it a little. How about, "Do unto *yourself* as you would have them do unto you?" Take care of yourself, too. You are as valuable as anyone else. You should not always be at the bottom of the list. You know we never get to the bottom.

Everyone knows that people respond better when we speak encouragingly to them. Do the same for yourself—treat yourself with love. Develop the habit of positive thinking about yourself.

Initiate your own Peace Plan by talking nicely to yourself. (You do talk to yourself, don't you?) Here are some examples of poisonous and encouraging comments:

Poisonous Talk	*Loving Talk*
I can't do as well as everybody else.	I'm unique! I do things differently than others.

Poisonous Talk	Loving Talk
I'll never get done on time. I might as well quit now.	I may not get this completed, but I am making progress.
Nobody likes what I do even when I do my best.	I don't know what they'll think of this, but I like it, and I can choose whether or how much to respond to others' opinions.
I never look like Miss America.	It's her job to look good, and she has professional help! (And I'll bet she has insecure days, too.)
I'm so nervous I can't think straight.	I'm really nervous, but I can take a deep breath and handle it. I always get through it.
I have so many things to do. I can't get them all done.	I have so many things to do. I'll make a list and decide what my priorities are and which I need to do. I don't have to do everything. I can choose.

Relaxation Techniques

Select a relaxation technique and incorporate it into your life—today, not tomorrow. Make time for yourself daily, even if you start with three minutes. That's three minutes when you do not have to answer the phone, speak to anyone, or do anything. Then double "your" time by making it happen twice a day.

People often tense their muscles as a reaction to stress. Muscle tension can be reduced. One technique I like simply has me focus my awareness on my body. As I sit at my desk or during a juice (not coffee) break or even when driving, I inhale and slowly observe or "scan" my body, searching out tense muscles. As I exhale, I relax the muscles that are tense. Sometimes when I'm scanning, I silently recite some phrase that has a calming effect, such as "serene and peaceful" or "quiet, calm."

I recorded a relaxation tape because many of my clients reported that listening to someone else's soothing voice helps them learn to relax. (See the Resource Appendix.) The classic work on the subject is *The Relaxation Response* by Herbert Benson.[1]

We have a name for focused relaxation, of course. Meditation is not some mystical practice. It is a natural way to quietly turn off the full complexity of life, to become calm in the midst of activity.

You have probably heard of active listening, listening carefully to what the other person is saying without judgment or interruption. Meditation is active listening to yourself. It is about quieting the mind, and then listening to it. Meditation is about living and enjoying the complexity and richness of each moment, not yesterday's happenings or tomorrow's projects.

Through meditation we learn to focus on the present moment. We learn what really interests and concerns us. Meditation teaches us to distance ourselves from emotional involvement in difficult situations. It's learning to be a human *being*, not a human *doing*.

For the best explanation and how-to book, pick up *Full Catastrophe Living: Using the Wisdom of Your Body and Mind to Face Stress, Pain, and Illness*, by Jon Kabat-Zinn, Ph.D.[2]

Massage

Another excellent way to relax is through massage. Chronic tension produces tightness in the musculature, causing a buildup of the waste and toxic by-products of cellular activity. According to the American Massage Therapy Association, increased circulation is one of the primary benefits of massage. This increase speeds the removal of these by-products and provides increased nutrients and oxygen to each cell.

Relaxation is a secondary effect of massage. During a massage, the body releases endorphins, natural painkillers produced by the body. (Endorphins are also released when we exercise.) As the muscles relax and loosen their grip on the body's soft tissue, the nerves become calmer. Energy flows more smoothly throughout the body.

Increased circulation and relaxation are two reasons why massage is so effective. Personally, I like it because it feels good.

Stress Relief from GABA

Many women find that GABA helps to relieve stress, anxiety, and depression.[3] GABA, Gamma Amino Butyric Acid, is a natural substance which concentrates its activity in the brain during the first part of the cycle and becomes more active in the reproductive cycle during the last half of the cycle. (This means that women are likely to feel more stressed during the last half of their cycle.) GABA supplements calm down our overreactions somewhat. It is not addictive. You'll find it in health food stores.

Coping with Stress

Here are ten tips for coping with stress. Which ones will you incorporate into your life? Start with one (that's not adding a lot of stress), and then include others which appeal to you.

1. Hang a "Do Not Disturb" sign on your door. Then read, exercise, nap, meditate.

2. Make time to visit a museum, church, or friend, or to browse in a bookstore.

3. Practice listening to others talk.

4. Do one thing at a time.

5. Write things down. Don't try to remember that dental appointment, gallon of milk, or who called.

6. Allow more time than you think you need to get to your appointments.

7. Be prepared to wait for everything—haircuts, appointments, kids, etc. I always keep something in the car that I want to read. Then I don't get upset when everything doesn't go according to my plan. I can get things done even while I'm waiting; or I can take advantage of the chance to relax.

8. Rid your environment of clutter. If you haven't worn it or used it for a year, give it away.

9. Listen to a stress reduction tape. (See Resource Appendix.)

10. Buy 1/4" self-sticking green dots. (You can find them in an office supply store. They are used to identify file folders.) Put them everywhere—on the bathroom mirror, the refrigerator, above the stove and sink, on the phone, on the rear view mirror and steering wheel in the car, on the microwave and the computer, everywhere. Then, every time you see one, take a deep breath and relax.

I invite you to take a one-minute break right now. Before you go to the next chapter, try the following mini-relaxation exercise. Read it, then close your eyes and do it. No fair peeking at the next chapter till you finish this one!

Envision yourself outside on a sunny day.

Blow as much air out of your lungs as possible three times.

Allow your legs to relax.

Allow your back, arms, and shoulders to relax.

Allow your chin to move toward your chest.

Allow your face and scalp to relax.

Put the book down, close your eyes, and listen to your heart beat for a full minute.

Relax. This is your time.

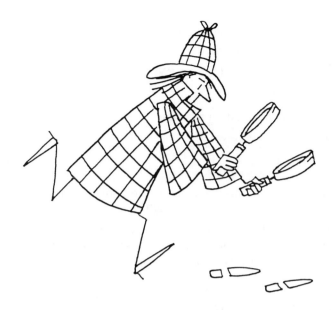

OTHER POSSIBLE CAUSES

PMS is not a traditional infectious disease or an organ failure. We can't take an antibiotic, an antidepressant, or a tranquilizer to get rid of the cause. PMS is an imbalance of the body's
systems. When we talk about the "causes" of PMS, we need to
keep this in mind. When we say that drinking too much caffeine
"causes" PMS, we really mean that caffeine increases PMS
symptoms and that eliminating it makes the symptoms less
severe.

With that in mind, let's go through a checklist of possible
PMS causes that we've already discussed.

- Thyroid system malfunction
- Caffeine
- Poor diet, especially one with sugar and NutraSweet
- Inadequate level of vitamins and minerals

- Possible estrogen-progesterone imbalance (not yet established)
- Sleep disorder (classic PMS)
- Inadequate light
- Atypical Candida albicans
- Lack of exercise
- Stress

If you have eliminated the above causes, but you still have symptoms, there are six other possible causes to address: 1) food sensitivities or allergies, 2) intestinal parasites, 3) environmental sensitivities, 4) mercury fillings, 5) exhausted adrenal glands, and 6) unresolved physical or sexual abuse. Let's discuss them briefly.

Food Sensitivities or Allergies

One of the women I worked with had incorporated all of the previous suggestions into her life. Much to her frustration, a vaginal yeast infection still appeared each time she had sex with her husband. So he started a Candida cleansing program. (Since men can also have Candida, he might have been reinfecting her.) He soon felt better himself, with a higher energy level, no more Candida-related symptoms (of which he had been unaware), and a five pound weight loss. That would usually stop a woman's vaginal infections. But this woman still got yeast infections.

After discussing her diet again in detail, I recommended that she go off all dairy products for ten days, then drink a glass of milk by itself. If there was no reaction within four days of elimination or reintroduction of the food, she could safely assume that she did not have a milk sensitivity. The process is called "eliminate and challenge." The idea is to eliminate the possible offending food for ten days and then challenge the body to respond to a single serving.

She stopped eating everything with dairy in it. She had a headache and some other symptoms on the third or fourth day. After that she felt better. When she reintroduced milk products, she immediately felt irritable and got a headache. She had an uncomfortable vaginal discharge the next day. Then she remembered that her mother had told her that she had been sensitive to milk as an infant. She had been eating milk, cheese, or yogurt daily.

The story has a happy ending. She made several changes to the family diet. For example, cheeseburgers are out, but she adds grilled onions. She puts guacamole instead of sour cream on tacos. They eat fruit for dessert instead of ice cream. The whole family feels better.

You may have been tested for food allergies in the past and nothing showed up. Unfortunately, although skin testing is reliable for inhalants such as house dust, dog and cat dander, and pollen, it is not reliable for food.

If you think a specific food may be causing you difficulty, try the eliminate and challenge test. If you don't feel well when you reintroduce the tested food, you have three choices: 1) leave it out of your diet and feel well, 2) eat small portions, infrequently, and feel some symptoms, or 3) eat all you want and have the same symptoms you do now.

Another woman reported that her children noticed a connection between erratic behavior on her part and green olives. She was astonished when her kids begged her not to eat even *one* olive. She remembered that the last time she ate olives she flew into a tirade. She decided that green olives weren't worth an emotional outburst.

The most common allergy-producing foods are dairy, wheat, soy, and corn. If you decide to do your own eliminate and challenge test, be sure to reintroduce or "challenge" your body with the freshest, purest form of the food. You don't want to avoid wheat and milk forever if your reaction was really caused by the preservatives in the bread or the food coloring in that processed cheese log.

I discovered that I have no reaction to dairy, wheat, or soybeans. Then I tried corn. I eliminated corn with no withdrawal symptoms. Then I challenged my body to respond by eating nearly a whole can of corn by itself. (I didn't want to guess later whether I had a reaction or not.) I was *very* unhappy when I became depressed and sleepy within 20 minutes. I couldn't stay awake. I was in tears, partly from the reaction and partly from the thought of never eating corn on the cob or popcorn again. My reaction was so clear-cut that I didn't eat corn for weeks. But when summer came, I decided that one ear of corn on the cob was worth depression later. So I ate it. Nothing happened! I tried other forms of corn. I could eat popcorn (if I made it myself), corn on the cob, and frozen corn. I ran into problems with corn chips and nachos; I could eat one brand but all the others gave me a headache. The labels on all the brands listed only corn, water and salt. Today I suspect that the preservatives in canned corn, microwave popcorn, and chips caused the reaction. Since I have a reaction to some highly processed foods, I made my choice. I skip canned corn, make my own popcorn, and eat chips just once in a while. (Chips aren't healthy food anyway.)

If you find that you are sensitive to something, eliminate it for six to 12 months. You may find that it doesn't bother you after that. Some people are able to gradually expand their diets to include a formerly offending food.

Candida can cause people to have an allergic reaction to foods to which they wouldn't otherwise be allergic. Remember that a Candida infection can allow large food particles to cross the intestinal wall (the condition known as "leaky gut.") Our bodies activate our immune systems to fight those interlopers. This creates an allergic response. The way we experience this response is largely determined by our genetic make-up. Some of us get aching joints, others get headaches, diarrhea, asthma, etc. To further complicate the picture, our reactions may not start for three to four days. With a delayed reaction, laboratory tests that are meant to detect food allergies are frequently inaccurate.

A detailed discussion of food sensitivities or allergies is beyond the scope of this book. A detailed discussion of food sensitivities and allergies is beyond the scope of this book. Dr. William Crook's *Are You Allergic?* is an excellent overview.[1] *Food Allergies,* by Neil S. Orenstein, Ph.D., and Sarah Bingham,

M.S., sets out an easily followed plan to help you uncover your own food allergies.[2] Jonathan Wright, M.D., has also written a very readable, informative book entitled *Dr. Wright's Book of Nutritional Therapy*.[3] For further information, check the Select Bibliography.[4,5,6]

Parasites

Some women take an unusually long time to recover from Candida. I then suspect microscopic intestinal parasites. Unfortunately, although we have many excellent laboratories in this country, most are not equipped to identify these parasitic and bacterial infections, just as they often miss Candida infections. A specialty lab must be used to identify the pathogens.[7] When the parasites, which are generating toxins, are eliminated, the individual feels wonderful.

Environmental Sensitivities

Sometimes women with atypical Candida develop heightened sensitivities to their environment.[8] Some women's symptoms worsen in the autumn when fallen leaves decay. Others find that their lungs hurt when they are exposed to perfume or tobacco smoke. I had to avoid perfume and cosmetic counters in department stores, and I instinctively held my breath when I walked down the detergent aisle at the grocery store.

Candida infections make some people hypersensitive to related molds and fungi, such as the mold growing in old houses or musty basements. I've known a handful of women who had to move—and then they stayed healthy.

Mercury Fillings

A 1989 study reported in the *American Journal of Psychotherapy* correlated silver amalgam tooth fillings with PMS, stress, poor memory, and fatigue.[9] Significant improvement was noted after the fillings were removed.

Silver amalgam tooth fillings contain mercury, a highly toxic metal. Each time we chew, a minute amount of mercury is released from these fillings. It accumulates in our cells. Although many people feel okay once their fillings are removed, the International and American Association of Clinical Nutritionists notes that others feel ill until the mercury is removed from their cells.

If your mouth is full of silver amalgam fillings, you may wish to consider mercury as a possible cause of your PMS. Unfortunately, filling removal is very delicate because the removal process itself releases mercury into the body. Some specialists prefer not to remove them for this reason. Please consult an up-to-date specialist before you decide to have your mercury fillings removed. You may also wish to read Sam Ziff's book, *Silver Dental Fillings: The Toxic Time Bomb,* or contact Dental Amalgam Mercury Syndrome (DAMS), Inc.[10,11]

Exhausted Adrenal Glands

Recent research is also turning up an increase in exhausted adrenal glands. This problem is particularly common in those with a malfunctioning thyroid system because their adrenals are struggling to get their thyroids to work properly.[12]

Physical and Sexual Abuse

Tragically, some women must deal with repressed or conscious but unresolved memories of sexual or physical abuse. These issues are extremely difficult to address but are worth the effort. When they are resolved, these women feel better physically, psychologically, emotionally, and spiritually. The historical *trauma* must become historical *fact*. Only then can purely physical remedies—cutting back on caffeine, exercising, etc.—be fully effective in relieving the symptoms of PMS.[13,14]

You may feel overwhelmed at this point in trying to uncover the reasons for your symptoms, especially since many people still think that PMS is a hormonal problem. After all, it does occur the last half of each cycle. And many women do feel better on natural progesterone because it calms the central nervous system. But remember the chapter on progesterone? Researchers have not yet established a correlation between the severity of symptoms and progesterone levels. Nor has anyone found a correlation between PMS and abnormal levels of progesterone and estrogen. Also, progesterone does not get rid of food cravings, insomnia, or migraines. Progesterone also stimulates Candida growth, which may have been the original problem.

Other people think that PMS, or Candida, is caused by hypoglycemia. A classic sign of hypoglycemia is that symptoms increase when a person has not eaten for a while. However, a Candida infection often causes a similar symptom pattern. The Candida multiply rapidly when blood sugar is high after eating. They begin to die and release their toxins when it drops. We have to study the individual's history or get a sophisticated lab test to be sure of the real cause.

Look in the next chapter. I think it will help you sort out the different causes so that *you* can put *your* puzzle back together.

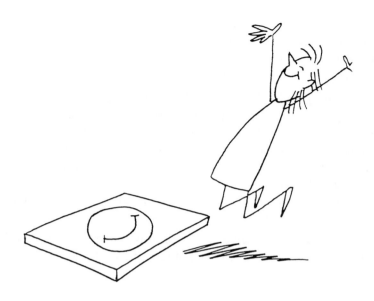

PUTTING THE PUZZLE TOGETHER

Let's review the sixteen possible causes of PMS that we have discussed:

- Thyroid system malfunction
- Caffeine
- Poor diet, especially one with sugar and NutraSweet
- Inadequate level of vitamins and minerals
- Possible estrogen-progesterone imbalance (not yet established)
- Sleep disorder (classic PMS)
- Inadequate light
- Atypical Candida albicans
- Lack of exercise
- Stress

- Food sensitivities or allergies
- Parasites
- Environmental sensitivities
- Mercury fillings
- Exhausted adrenal glands
- Unresolved physical or sexual abuse

Where do you start to put your PMS puzzle together? You've already started. Reading this book is the first step.

Remember the saying, "Knowledge is power?" The goal of this book is to add to what you already know. You know your body and your medical history better than anyone. Now you need to hear that it is difficult, but not impossible, to help yourself.

You can decide to eliminate caffeine and NutraSweet (aspartame) and to choose a diet which will help you regain your health. You can eliminate or sharply reduce sugar consumption. You can take those important vitamins and minerals.

Get outside in the original full spectrum light whenever you can. Avoid burning, of course. Use full spectrum ultraviolet-producing lights indoors even on sunny summer days, since the glass windows in houses, cars, and offices block ultraviolet light.

Get a full night's sleep in a darkened room. Get off the couch and exercise, outside when possible. Ask for help or find some way to reduce your stress load. Please contact a counselor or spiritual advisor if you suspect abuse. Those memories can be rough, and it's good to be with a professional as you recover your inner strength.

Let your husband, your family, and your friends support you. They can help you identify possible food sensitivities, help you reduce your stress levels, find a way to let you sleep enough, and give invaluable moral support. Remember, PMS isn't just "in your head." It's okay to ask for support, although you *can* do it alone. By sharing your journey back to health, you might even inspire a friend or relative to conquer her own PMS!

Your doctor or other health care practitioner is your ally. He or she can coach you through the transition back to health. Your doctor may wish to run laboratory tests for hypoglycemia, Candida, parasites, estrogen, and progesterone. If a blood test reveals hypoglycemia, you may wish to read *Hypoglycemia: A Better Approach* by Airola.[1] Vitamin and mineral levels can be determined by other tests. Your doctor can also help you if your body temperature test indicates you may need thyroid supplementation.

As you have noticed, I include physicians and other health care providers in the quest to help people. I reject the term "alternative medicine" because that connotes an either/or approach to health and healing. I prefer "complementary medicine" and "holistic medicine." These recognize that the best approach is to take advantage of both traditional healing wisdom and the technology offered by conventional medicine.

Let's look again at the three main undetected causes of PMS, which are closely intertwined and often overlooked: undetected thyroid system malfunction, classic PMS, and atypical Candidiasis. Mark the items that apply to you.

Thyroid System Malfunction

Note: Thyroid blood test may be normal.

_____ Family history of thyroid malfunction

_____ Always cold, or cold hands and feet

_____ Difficulty losing weight

_____ Skin turns yellow in response to high intake of beta carotene (instead of converting it to vitamin A)

_____ Poor immune system function and frequent illness

Classic PMS

_____ Severe symptoms at ovulation and before menstruation

_____ Poor sleep patterns from ovulation until menstrual flow starts

_____ Family history of alcohol abuse or migraines

_____ Personal or family history of sleep disorders, such as:
     trouble going to sleep
     trouble staying asleep
     sleeping long hours
     walking, talking or grinding teeth while sleeping
     childhood bedwetting

_____ Noticeable mood or energy changes which correlate with the amount of full spectrum light

_____ Salt and/or sugar cravings

Atypical Candidiasis

History of

_____ Antibiotics

_____ Birth control pills

_____ Pregnancy

_____ Steroids (cortisone, Prednisone)

Contributing factors

_____ High stress

_____ Poor diet

_____ Living in an area with high humidity

_____ Living or working in a moldy building

Health history

_____ Frequent respiratory infections

_____ Irritable Bowel Syndrome (IBS)

_____ Vaginal infections

_____ Adult onset acne

_____ Unexplained muscle aches or joint aches

_____ Headaches, migraines

_____ Urinary tract infections (UTI)

Atypical Candidiasis (cont'd)

Hallmarks

_____ Sugar cravings

_____ Symptoms worse on damp days or in moldy buildings

_____ Symptoms better, then worse, after eating carbohydrates

If several checks appear under one symptom heading, reread the chapters which discusses that cause. You may have identified a piece of your PMS puzzle.

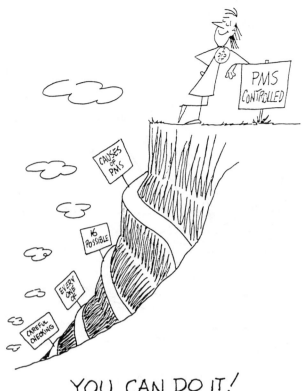

YOU CAN DO IT!

From my experience, I can state very positively that *you do not have to have PMS*. It may take time and effort, but it can be done.

Remember the poster in my office:

"You are never given a wish without also being given

the power to make it come true.

You may have to work for it, however."

– Richard Bach
Illusions

Always keep in mind that there is at least *one* reason for what you are experiencing. With persistence you, too, can get your PMS under control. Your puzzle can be put together.

Believe in yourself.

You *can* get well.

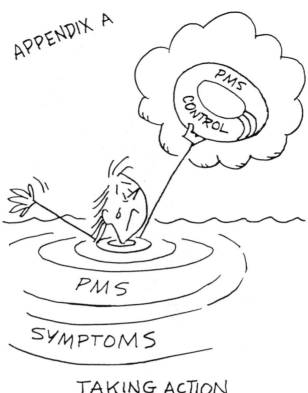

TAKING ACTION

Comments for Families and Friends

Identifying the causes of PMS is only the first step. The woman with PMS then has to make the changes in her diet and lifestyle that will help her body heal itself. Her family and friends are crucial in supporting these changes. It is extremely important that she not feel alone.

Several years ago I asked my women's support group what they would like me to tell their friends, families, and doctors. It was as if I had opened a fire hydrant—they overwhelmed me and my secretary for the next two hours. They told me:

> *"PMS anger feels different inside. When I get angry, it wells up from the inside. It's like a thermometer, like a champagne bottle that's been shaken up."*

"The symptoms are overwhelming to me and scare me. I feel a superhuman strength. I know that I'm not a wild, violent person; inside, I'm a pacifist."

"Sometimes what I say is unnerving to me, too. It's not a personal attack."

"When I go into a rage, please hug me tight. I'm terrified, I don't trust myself, I'm so scared. Please stay with me. I know it's not easy for you. It's not easy for me either. Then let me cry, or cry with me."

"Help me understand it. After an episode, tell me that it's a disease. It's so discouraging to live with this. So often I feel that I've got it under control, and then it hits me again."

"Plan with me when I'm well what the best way to deal with PMS would be. Acknowledge how I feel. Maybe you could say, 'I see you're having a bad day.' You might ask what you could do. I probably won't know, but I will be aware that you care and that you asked."

"I get so tired of taking care of myself."

"I can understand that you would like to leave sometimes. I don't like to live with me either."

"When all I can do is cry, just tell me that you love me. I may deny it and question it and tell you that you couldn't, that you're just feeling sorry for me, but deep inside, I'll hear you."

"We have a good sex life the first part of the cycle, but premenstrually I'm really not interested. I know it hurts him when I feel that way. I don't understand it, either."

"Before my period I go into a world like mental illness—crying jags, phobias about people and things around me. It's like impending doom. I constantly think about dying. Then my period comes and I'm singing again."

> *"After a particularly severe episode, please take over for me. I probably can't even tell you, but to recuperate I need to be alone with no responsibilities."*

> *"It's so frustrating. During my good days, I bowl 200; during the bad days, I average 110."*

> *"I feel as if I'm in a dark hole and I'll never get out."*

> *"Tell them that we're sorry that our illness affects them."*

> *"Sometimes just the sound and movement of other people bother me and I need to withdraw."*

> *"Recovery is a long road. Please don't think I'm fine when I'm halfway there. I still need your understanding and your help."*

And the most important thing that these women pleaded with me to say is:

> *"It's real. It's real. Tell them it's real!"*

While You're Getting Better

Most women with PMS tell me that the physical symptoms make them feel miserable, but the really bad part is the effect of PMS on their emotions. Still, no matter how bad they are feeling, women with PMS know that they are responsible for their actions.

Many women find that it is easier to deal with the emotional roller coaster of PMS once they know that it can be overcome. For many women, doing something about their PMS—eating better, taking supplements, exercising, adding full spectrum light to their homes and offices, paying more attention to sleep patterns, learning to take time for themselves, even reading a book about how they will feel better—helps them feel more in control of their lives right away. It often makes them less depressed and less stressed. This alone helps their minds and bodies deal with the PMS better. They can become healthy!

Dealing with Emotions

Women and their families know that PMS affects everyone. Sometimes family members are the victims of a PMS outburst; sometimes they are the instigators. Some family problems are related to PMS and others are not. I use the example of Dirty Socks: A woman with PMS may explode in anger at a pair of dirty socks left on the floor. At that moment she may feel that *everyone* is irresponsible except her and that she has to do all the work. Or she may dissolve in tears because others don't seem to do their share of the work. She may feel like a failure as a mother since she has not taught the family members to put their dirty socks in the clothes basket. She may feel like a slave if she feels she has to pick up after family members. None of the above responses are appropriate. She has overreacted. But the dirty socks are still on the floor. The socks should be picked up at that moment, but the family must wait until she has calmed down and is logical again to address the issue. They may have to wait until after her period starts. As she regains her health, the dirty socks resume their proper importance as an issue to be resolved. Family interaction is not "me-vs.-them," it's "we're-all-in-this-together."

Many times, after the PMS is under control, issues which produced anger may need to be addressed. Justified anger is not wrong or a weakness. It is an emotional response to a perceived injustice. Anger may be expressed as mild irritation or it may be an explosion. Either way, we need to learn appropriate ways of dealing with our anger. These do not include smiling through our tears, playing the martyr, keeping a stiff upper lip, or finding a victim and exploding in rage. Though it is difficult to change patterns of behavior, remember that a martyr never does anything to change.

Anger management and control does not mean anger suppression. As a woman with PMS regains her health, she can learn to express her anger with carefully chosen words. As I was growing up, I was often reminded, "It's not what you say, it's how you say it." You may choose to draw a picture or write an angry letter, but don't deliver it.

Anger may be an expression of fear or sadness or stress. Learn to say, "I get angry when ----." Look into your past experiences. Did something that happened yesterday, or a decade ago, trigger today's angry response?

Instead of asking "Why?" which can be demanding, practice asking "Would you explain it to me?" It's also okay to say, "I don't understand." Often that phrase enlists others' support, even a boss'. Both of you then have the chance to get the expectations clear.[1]

In *The Dance of Anger*, Harriet Goldhor Lerner explains that we learn to respond in a set pattern to another's usual way of acting and speaking, thus creating our own dance steps.[2] For example, when Grandma asks if the family is coming over for dinner on Sunday, you may get angry because you feel she's telling you what to do and implying that you're not a good mother to your children, that you don't know how to feed and care for them. But she may have entirely different motives. Perhaps Grandma invited you because she was taught that this is how a good grandmother should act. She might prefer to ask someone else over or even not have company. Or she might be asking because she wants to give you a break from cooking. If you don't express your feelings, neither of you will know how the other one feels. The relationship will hold resentment on both sides. When you change your response, your dance partner will necessarily change his or her dance steps too.

Are you familiar with the Serenity Prayer?

> God grant me Serenity
> To accept the things I cannot change,
> Courage to change the things I can,
> And Wisdom to know the difference.

It's a put-down to describe all of a woman's moods as PMS. All family members have moods. The women I know would much rather interact positively than deal with PMS and its emotional upheaval and physical symptoms.

As one doctor explained, "Having moods is not an illness. Being premenstrual is not an illness. Having severe premenstrual symptoms is an illness." One that can be overcome.

Support from Family and Friends

When she's crying, offer her a hug and a snack of whole grain crackers, popcorn, or an apple. If she's angry, gently suggest that she work off some of the anger by working out. Just taking a fast walk will help lower her adrenalin. She may need you to go with her to get her out the door, or she may need to go alone.

Support her in overcoming her PMS. Suggest that she fill out the questionnaires in this book. Then help her implement her chosen program. Remember that low self-confidence and low self-esteem are part of PMS. She will probably get discouraged and feel as if she'll never be her old self again. She'll need someone to coax her into starting again. She may need help finding a professional who understands thyroid system malfunction, atypical Candida, and serotonin/melatonin fluctuations. Help her prevent crises by lovingly suggesting that she eat little meals often. Take walks with her, or play catch or Frisbee. Surround her with full spectrum lights. Help her make time to listen to a stress reduction tape. Those are healthy physical and relationship habits to continue for a lifetime.

Be patient. She *will* get better, but it takes time. Then every-one will feel better.

The women in my support group asked me to please give their families this *very* important message:

> "*Most of all tell them that we love them. The way we act in a PMS crisis has nothing to do with the fact that we love them.*"

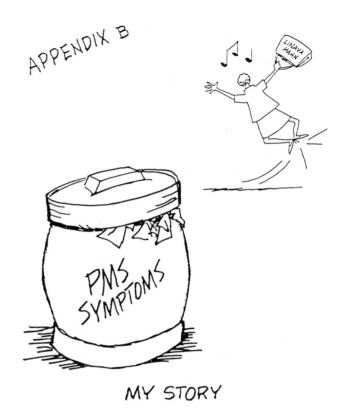

APPENDIX B

MY STORY

Hindsight tells me that I've had PMS since I started my periods. As a teen, I had a little bloating and cramps, a little breast tenderness, no big deal. In my 20s, I cried on Tuesday and got my period on Wednesday. Rather handy, really, because I'd know when to carry tampons and pads. I was basically quite healthy. I married, had two wonderful sons, and took birth control pills for ten years. In my mid-30s, I had a tubal ligation and my world fell apart.

Was I the happy, confident mom and school board president, or was I really unhappy and incompetent? My answer to myself depended on when I asked it. Some days, I couldn't think clearly. I cried at commercials on television. (Remember the phone company's "Reach out and touch someone" commercials?) Some days my muscles ached so badly that I could hardly get out of bed. My breasts hurt too much to take my bra off. I thought, "If this is what it's like to be mid-30s, I could skip the mid-60s."

Today I'm looking forward to my healthy, happy mid-60s and mid-90s and beyond.

Part of the month I enjoyed my inquisitive, enthusiastic children; the other part I thought they were messy and noisy. Even my cooking patterns changed. Sometimes I was creative; other times I had to ask the kids if we should have pizza or spaghetti for dinner. Fortunately, I could still turn on the oven or boil water. I just couldn't decide which! My husband didn't know what to do with me and my PMS symptoms, so he withdrew, a not uncommon reaction.

Was I impossible to get along with or was I too tolerant? Which one was the real me? It was very scary. I was afraid I was going crazy. I joked about reserving a room for myself in the psychiatric ward of the hospital for 17 days a month. The other week (I had a short cycle), I was too happy and busy to think of hospitalization. I was cooking, cleaning, running errands, paying bills, having fun with the kids, and doing volunteer work in the schools.

The intermittent timing of my symptoms was a definite clue: I felt fine one week and predictably miserable for more than two weeks. But I hadn't recognized the pattern yet.

With my sons in high school, I had time to do anything I wanted. What I did was go back to bed. I just lay there. I didn't even read or turn over. I was too exhausted. I didn't know what had happened to my good spirits and high energy. It was a big day when I could get the jeans and underwear washed. I couldn't do the colored clothes. I couldn't decide which were light-colored and which were dark-colored!

There were times when I would enthusiastically run an international student committee meeting and cheerfully wave good-bye as I drove off. Then I would pull into the next driveway and cry for 15 minutes because I didn't know where I would find the energy to drive home.

Fortunately, about that time I saw a television talk show which described symptoms like mine. Maybe I was normal after all! Hope returned. I kept track of my bad days on a calendar.

Sure enough, they happened just before my period. Great! But wait. Maybe I just made that happen because I wanted an answer. Maybe it wasn't true. I stopped charting. Would the "nasties" appear if I didn't know when my period was coming? They did. When my flow started, I could look back at the previous difficult days. My PMS diagnosis was confirmed. (Even today, charting is the most accurate way of diagnosing PMS.)

Now that I knew what I had, what could I do to feel better? That's when my quest for information started. I knew what it was like to be healthy all month because my PMS was not severe when I was a teen. Those memories of a healthier self inspired me to solve the puzzle and regain my health.

As you know by now, PMS is a complicated disorder to treat. In addition, many of the advances in PMS care are very recent and are being made in different fields, in conventional and holistic medicine, psychology, and nutrition. I found that, in order to develop a comprehensive PMS control program, I needed to work with experts from all over the world and study original research.

Once I solved my own PMS puzzle, I found that other women with PMS asked me for information. Fortunately, a lot more is known today than when I started my search for health. That is why I wrote this book.

PMS is a puzzle with several pieces. What took me years to learn and apply can now be put together in a matter of months. Recovery can start the first month. You simply need to find the missing pieces of your PMS puzzle and fill them in or correct them.

Good luck!

APPENDIX C. RESOURCE APPENDIX

The Importance of Vitamins and Minerals

Nutritional surveys reported out in both the U.S. and Canada within the last five years have demonstrated an embarrassing number of people in both countries with measurable malnutrition of one kind or another, particularly relating to certain vitamins and minerals. I say embarrassing because we have the knowledge and other kinds of resources necessary to prevent this kind of disorder, and yet even a conservative estimate of the number of cases in the United States would get into the millions.[1]

–Dr. Virgil Wodicka, Food & Drug
Administration

Like physical fitness or thyroid function, vitamin deficiency is not a yes-or-no occurrence. One study postulates five stages of increasing vitamin deficiency.[2] Please note stage three.

1. Reduction in tissue stores with decreased urinary excretion.

2. Reduced enzyme activity due to decreased coenzyme with minimal urinary excretion.

3. Behavioral effects become evident, including insomnia, somnolence, irritability, adverse psychological competency scores, lack of appetite, decrease in weight, and decreased immune system competence.

4. Classical deficiency state, like scurvy.

5. Death.

Where to Find It:

Nutritional Supplements and Other Products

Acidophilus powder or capsules
Evening Primrose Oil and Omega-3 and Omega-6 products
Microcrystalline Hydroxyapatite (highly absorbable calcium)
PMS Information and Relaxation Tape
Today anti-stress multivitamin/mineral supplement, designed for
    women with PMS
PMS Control Kit—Information and Relaxation Tape, *Today*
    antistress multivitamin/mineral, and acidophilus, with or
    without *PMS: Solving the Puzzle* book

Full Spectrum Light Products

Full spectrum light boxes, fluorescent tubes, incandescent
(standard) bulbs, and full spectrum transmitting sunglasses
    Call Light for Health at 800 468-1104

Full spectrum transmitting hard contacts
    Call Contact Lens Supply at 800 833-7525
    and ask for the PMMA lens

Natural Progesterone and/or Natural Estrogen

    Call Bajamar Pharmaceutical Co. at 800 255-8025

Progestone-HP (extract of wild yam cream)

    Call the Dixie PMS Center at 800 767-9232

See the last page of the book for an order form for mail orders.

Sample Insurance Claim Letter

Re:
Policy #

Dear Claims Adjuster:

This letter explains why a full-spectrum, radiation-shielded light box has been recommended and prescribed for _____. A large and growing body of medical research shows that premenstrual syndrome (PMS), as well as Seasonal Affective Disorder (SAD), are linked to the amount and type of light which enters our eyes and regulates serotonin and melatonin levels.

These conditions have been shown in many studies in both the United States and Europe to respond to treatment with phototherapy. As stated in an abstract in the September 1989 *American Journal of Psychiatry*, "Bright light may offer an alternative to the pharmacologic treatment of premenstrual mood disorders." Our experience shows that to be true. According to the December 8, 1993 issue of the *Journal of the American Medical Association* (JAMA), "For many patients with SAD, light therapy should be regarded as first-line treatment, given its high success and acceptance rate." (Vol. 270, no. 22, pages 2717-20)

The application of phototherapy is recent but no longer considered experimental. Numerous medical journal articles describe the treatment and the physiology behind it. In order to administer phototherapy *adequately*, a full spectrum light box is medically necessary and preferable to other forms of treatment.

It is our experience and continuing expectation that the one-time cost of the light box improves the overall health of the patient. Light boxes lower insurance costs by reducing the number of visits to doctors' offices as well as lowering the dose and cost of some prescription medication.

Sincerely,

Citations for Insurance Letter

B. L. Parry MD, S. L. Berga MD, N. Mostofi et al., "Morning Versus Evening Treatment of Late Luteal Phase Dysphoric Disorder;" *American Journal of Psychiatry* 146:9 (Sept. 1989): pp. 1215-17.

B. L. Parry MD, S. L. Berga MD, D. F. Kripke MD, et al., "Altered Waveform of Plasma Nocturnal Melatonin Secretion in Premenstrual Depression," *Archives of General Psychiatry* 47 (1991): pp. 1139-46.

B. L. Parry MD, N. E. Rosenthal MD, L. Tamarkin, & T. Wehr, "Treatment of a Patient with Seasonal Premenstrual Syndrome," *American Journal of Psychiatry* 144, no. 6 (June 1987): pp. 762-66.

A. J. Rapkin MD, E. Edelmuth MD, L. C. Chang, et al., "Whole-Blood Serotonin in Premenstrual Syndrome," *Obstetrics and Gynecology* 70, no. 4 (Oct. 1987): pp. 533-37.

C. Thompson, D. Stinson, & A. Smith, "Seasonal Affective Disorder and Season-Dependent Abnormalities of Melatonin Suppression by Light," *Lancet* 336 (1990): pp. 703-6.

ORDER FORM

We have included an order form because it would be a disservice to give you information on how to control PMS without giving you a place to obtain the products you need. Products and prices change over time, so it is impractical to include a complete product and price list. We will add new items as our research and your requests indicate. We pledge to offer the highest quality products at the lowest possible prices. We have included some product information in the Resource Appendix. For up-to-date information, or to order by telephone, call 800 520-3822.

Product:_____Quantity _____

_____Quantity _____

_____Quantity _____

Ordered by:

Name _____

Address _____

City _____

State/Province _____ Zip/Postal Code _____

Daytime Phone (_____) _____

Ship to (if different from above):

Name _____

Address _____

City _____State____Zip _____

Method of Payment

☐ VISA   ☐ MasterCard   ☐ Check or Money Order

Card Number _____ Exp. Date _____

Name on card _____

Signature _____

SELECT BIBLIOGRAPHY

GENERAL BACKGROUND INFORMATION
–PMS

L. H. Back, "Identifying the Etiologies of Physiologically-based Mood Disorders and their Related Clinical Implications," *Women and Therapy* 12 (1992): pp. 137-50.

M. Harrison, *Self-help for Premenstrual Syndrome* (New York: Random House, 1982).

S. Lark, *Premenstrual Syndrome Self-help Book: A Woman's Guide to Feeling Good All Month* (Los Angeles: Forman, 1984).

C. Northrup, *Women's Bodies, Women's Wisdom: Creating Physical and Emotional Health and Healing* (New York: Bantam, 1994).

P. M. S. O'Brien, *Premenstrual Syndrome* (Oxford: Blackwell Scientific, 1987).

R. L. Reid, "Premenstrual Syndrome," *New England Journal of Medicine* 324, no. 17 (Apr. 25, 1991): pp. 1208-10.

D. R. Rubinow, "The Premenstrual Syndrome: New Views," *Journal of the American Medical Association* 268, no. 14 (Oct. 14, 1992): pp. 1908-12.

–NUTRITION

N. Angier, "Vitamins Win Support as Potent Agents of Health," *New York Times* (Mar. 10, 1992): p. C1.

J. F. Balch and P. A. Balch, *Prescription for Nutritional Healing* (Garden City Park, NY: Avery, 1990).

E. M. Haas, *Staying Healthy with Nutrition: The Complete Guide to Diet & Nutritional Medicine* (Berkeley, CA: Celestial Arts, 1992).

"The New Scoop on Vitamins," *Time* (Apr. 6, 1992): pp 54-59.

M. R. Werback, *Nutritional Influences on Illness: A Sourcebook of Clinical Research* (New Canaan, CT: Keats, 1988).

M. R. Werback, *Nutritional Influences on Illness: A Sourcebook of Clinical Research [Supplemental Chapters]* (Tarzana, CA: Third Line, 1991): pp. S12-S23.

CHAPTER 3. THE BASICS

1. J. FF. Watts, W. R. Butt, R. L. Edwards, & G. Holder, "Hormonal Studies in Women with Premenstrual Tension," *British Journal of Obstetrics and Gynaecology* 92 (March 1985): pp. 247-55.
   Ovulation may occur 16-17 days before menstruation.

CHAPTER 5. DO YOU HAVE PMS?

1. D. F. Horrobin, "The Role of Essential Fatty Acids and Prostaglandins in the Premenstrual Syndrome," *Journal of Reproductive Medicine* 28, no. 7 (July 1983): pp. 465-68.
2. J. Puolakka et al., "Biochemical and Clinical Effects of Treating the Premenstrual Syndrome with Prostaglandin Synthesis Precursors," *Journal of Reproductive Medicine* 30, no. 3 (March 1985): pp. 149-53.
3. J. Graham, *Evening Primrose Oil* (New York: Thorsons, 1984): pp. 36-41.
4. Ibid., p. 29.

5. S. Lark, *Premenstrual Syndrome Self-Help Book: A Woman's Guide to Feeling Good All Month* (Los Angeles: Forman, 1984).

CHAPTER 7. THYROID SYSTEM MALFUNCTION

1. N. Brayshaw and D. D. Brayshaw, "Thyroid Hypofunction in Premenstrual Syndrome," (letter to the editor), *New England Journal of Medicine* 315, no. 23 (Dec. 4, 1986): pp. 1486-87.

2. N. Brayshaw, "PMS and Thyroid Dysfunction: Preliminary Research Reveals a Possible Connection," *PMS Access* 13 (May/June 1987): pp. 1-3.

3. N. Brayshaw, quoted in K. McCleary, "PMS, Insomnia...or Thyroid?" *American Health* 4 (Sept. 1985): p. 76.

4. B. Barnes, "The Treatment of Menstrual Disorders in General Practice," *Arizona Medicine* 6, no. 1 (Jan. 1949): pp. 33-34.

5. B. Barnes and L. Galton, *Hypothyroidism: The Unsuspected Illness* (New York: Harper & Row, 1976).

6. R. T. Golan, "Yeast Overgrowth." From the manuscript of *Optimal Wellness* (New York: Ballantine, pub. pending 1995): p. 2.

7. B. Barnes and L. Galton, *Hypothyroidism: The Unsuspected Illness* (New York: Harper & Row, 1976): pp. 128-30.

8. D. Nolan, *Ending Fatigue and Depression* (Redmond, WA: James, McCormick, 1987): pp. 54-60.

9. J. J. Haggerty, Jr. et al., "Subclinical Hypothyroidism: A Modifiable Risk Factor for Depression?" *American Journal of Psychiatry* 150, no. 3 (Mar. 1993): pp. 508-10.

10. B. Barnes and L. Galton, *Hypothyroidism: The Unsuspected Illness* (New York: Harper & Row, 1976).

11. Broda Barnes Research Foundation, P.O. Box 98, Trumbull, CT 06611. Phone 203 261-2101.

12. E. D. Wilson, *Wilson's Syndrome: The Miracle of Feeling Well* (Orlando, FL: Cornerstone, 1991).

13. A. R. Gaby, *Hypothyroidism: The Unsuspected Illness* (Audiotape) (Baltimore: AHMA Books, 1993).

14. B. Barnes and L. Galton, *Hypothyroidism: The Unsuspected Illness.* (New York: Harper & Row, 1976): pp. 42-48.

15. E. D. Wilson, *Wilson's Syndrome: The Miracle of Feeling Well* (Orlando, FL: Cornerstone, 1991).

16. A. R. Gaby, *Hypothyroidism: The Unsuspected Illness* (Audiotape) (Baltimore: AHMA Books, 1993).

17. B. Barnes and L. Galton, *Hypothyroidism: The Unsuspected Illness.* (New York: Harper & Row, 1976): pp. 42-48.

18. Broda Barnes Research Foundation, P.O. Box 98, Trumbull, CT 06611. Phone 203 261-2101.

19. Wright/Gaby Nutrition Institute, P.O. Box 21535, Baltimore, MD 21208. Their research library contains more than 23,000 scientific papers related to nutrition and natural medicine.

20. A. R. Gaby, *Hypothyroidism: The Unsuspected Illness* (Audiotape) (Baltimore: AHMA Books, 1993).

21. A. R. Gaby and D. S. Cooper, "Treatment with Thyroid Hormone," letter to the editor, *Journal of the American Medical Association* 262, no. 13 (Oct. 6, 1989): pp. 1773-74.

22. S. E. Langer and J. F. Scheer, *Solved: The Riddle of Illness* (New Canaan, CT: Keats, 1984).

23. V. J. M. Pop et al., "Postpartum Thyroid Dysfunction and Depression in an Unselected Population" (letter to the editor), *New England Journal of Medicine* 324, no. 25 (June 20, 1991): pp. 1815-16.

CHAPTER 8. *CAFFEINE*

1. 12 oz. Coke Classic = 40.5 grams (10 tsp.) sugar. Coca-Cola Consumer Information, P.O. Box 1734, Atlanta, GA 30301. Phone 800 438-2653.

2. K. Griffin, "Good News for Java Junkies," *Hippocrates* (Nov./Dec. 1989): pp. 18-22.

3. Ibid., p. 20.

4. P. W. Budoff, *No More Menstrual Cramps and Other Good News* (New York: G. P. Putnam's Sons, 1980): p. 93.

5. Ibid., p. 93.

6. M. L. Bunker and M. McWilliams, "Caffeine Content of Common Beverages," *Journal of the American Dietetic Association* 74 (Jan. 1979): pp. 28-32.

7. "Caffeine: How to Consume Less," *Consumer Reports* (Oct. 1981): pp. 597-99.

8. Sweetlite Natural Fructose Sugar, TKI Foods, P.O. Box 30, Swarthmore, PA 19081.

9. A. Sanchez et al., "Role of Sugars in Human Neutrophilic Phagocytosis," *American Journal of Clinical Nutrition* 26 (Nov. 1973): pp. 1180-84.

10. G. J. Oettle, P. M. Emmett, & K. W. Heaton, "Glucose and Insulin Responses to Manufactured and Whole-Food Snacks," *American Journal of Clinical Nutrition* 45, no. 1 (Jan. 1987): pp. 86-91.

11. "Grounds for Breaking the Coffee Habit? Avoiding Caffeine Eases Premenstrual Tension," *Tufts University Diet and Nutrition Letter* 7, no. 12 (Feb. 1990): Special Report, p. 5.

12. C. W. Bales, "Nutritional Aspects of Osteoporosis: Recommendations for the Elderly at Risk," *Annual Review of Gerontology and Geriatrics* 9 (1989): pp. 7-34 (caffeine p. 22).

13. M. Hernandez-Avila et al., "Caffeine, Moderate Alcohol Intake, and Risk of Fractures of the Hip and Forearm in Middle-Aged Women," *American Journal of Clinical Nutrition* 54 (1991): pp. 157-63.

CHAPTER 9. *WHAT ABOUT DIET?*

1. Healthy Mediterranean Diet Pyramid, developed by the Harvard School of Public Health, Oldways Preservation & Exchange Trust, and the World Health Organization European Regional Office. More in N. H. Jenkins, *The Mediterranean Diet Cookbook: A Delicious Alternative for Lifelong Health* (New York: Bantam, 1994).

2. J. D. Beasley and J. Swift, *The Kellogg Report: The Impact of Nutrition, Environment and Lifestyle on the Health of Americans* (Annandale-on-Hudson, New York: The Institute of Health Policy and Practice of The Bard College Center, 1989).

3. B. L. Smith, "Organic Foods vs. Supermarket Foods: Element Levels," *Journal of Applied Nutrition* 45 (1993): pp. 35-39.

4. F. E. Baer, "Why Organic Food Matters," *The Journal of Sustainable Agriculture* (Feb. 1989): p. 3.

5. E. C. G. Grant, "Food Allergies and Migraine," *Lancet* 1, no. 6495 (May 5, 1979): pp. 966-69.

6. E. S. Johnson, N. P. Kadam, D. M. Hylands, & P. J. Hylands, "Efficacy of Feverfew as Prophylactic Treatment of Migraine," *British Medical Journal* 291, no. 6495 (Aug. 31, 1985): pp. 569-73.

7. J. J. Murphy, S. Heptinstall, & J. R. A. Mitchell, "Randomised Double-Blind Placebo-Controlled Trial of Feverfew in Migraine Prevention," *Lancet* 2, no. 8604 (July 23, 1988): pp. 189-92.

8. C. Igram and J. Gray, *Eat Right to Live Long*, 5th ed. (Cedar Rapids, IA: Literary Visions, 1989).

9. W. Dufty, *Sugar Blues* (New York: Warner, 1975).

CHAPTER 10. VITAMINS AND MINERALS—YES OR NO?

1. L. Chaitow, "Understanding Alternative Medicine" (audiotape), *Alternative Medicine: The Definitive Guide* (Puyallup, WA: Future Medicine, 1993).

2. S. Lieberman and N. Bruning, *The Real Vitamin and Mineral Book* (Garden City Park, NY: Avery, 1990).

3   National Capital Poison Center

4. A. Frustaci et al., "Myocardial Magnesium Content, Histology, and Antiarrhythmic Response to Magnesium Infusion" (letter), *Lancet* 2, no. 8566 (Oct. 31, 1987): p. 1019.

5. C. J. M. van Tiggelen, J. P. C. Peperkamp, and J. F. W. Tertoolen, "Vitamin B$_{12}$ Levels of Cerebrospinal Fluid in Patients with Organic Mental Disorder," *Journal of Orthomolecular Psychiatry* 12 (1983): p. 305.

6. *Medical World News* 34, no. 1 (Jan. 1993): pp. 24-32, cited by R. A. Anderson in preconference workshop, American Holistic Medical Association Conference, Feb. 13-15, 1994, Seattle, WA.

7. C. Perlmutter and T. Hanlon, "Why Top Doctors Take Supplements (And Why You Should Know What They're Thinking...and Doing)," *Prevention* 46, no. 2 (Feb. 1994): p. 65.

8. W. Barr, "Pyridoxine Supplements in the Premenstrual Syndrome," *Practitioner* 228 (April 1984): pp. 425-27.

9. M. J. Williams, R. I. Harris, and B. C. Dean, "Controlled Trial of Pyridoxine in Premenstrual Syndrome," *Journal of International Medical Research* 13 (1985): pp. 174-79.

10. P. W. Adams et al., "Effect of Pyridoxine Hydrochloride Upon Depression Associated with Oral Contraception," *Lancet* 1, no. 7809 (April 28, 1973): pp. 897-904.

11. R. A. Sherwood et al., "Magnesium and the Premenstrual Syndrome," *Annals of Clinical Biochemistry* 23, no. 6 (Nov. 1986): pp. 667-70.

12. F. Facchinetti et al., "Oral Magnesium Successfully Relieves Premenstrual Mood Changes," *Obstetrics and Gynecology* 78, no. 2 (Aug. 1991): pp. 177-81.

13. O. Johnell et al., "Age and Sex Patterns of Hip Fracture—Changes in 30 Years," *Acta Orthopaedica Scandinavica* 55 (1984): pp. 290-92.

14. L. Cohen and R. Kitzes, "Infrared Spectroscopy and Magnesium Content of Bone Mineral in Osteoporotic Women," *Israeli Journal of Medical Sciences* 17 (1981): pp. 1123-25.

15. *Medical Tribune* (July 22, 1993): p. 1, cited by R. A. Anderson in preconference workshop, American Holistic Medical Association Conference, Feb. 13-15, 1994, Seattle, WA.

Of 31 women taking 250-750 mg magnesium daily for two years, 75% achieved bone mineral density increases of 1-8%. 17 women refusing the supplement had bone mineral losses of 1-3%.

16. F. H. Nielsen, C. D. Hunt, L. M. Mullen, & J. R. Hunt, *Effect of Dietary Boron on Mineral, Estrogen and Testosterone Metabolism in Postmenopausal Women* (Grand Forks, ND: U. S. Department of Agriculture, Agricultural Research Service, Grand Forks Human Nutrition Research Center): pp. 394-97.

Boron markedly reduced urinary excretion of calcium and magnesium in all women and even more so in the magnesium deficient women. Boron decreased phosphorus excretion in magnesium deficient women but not in magnesium-adequate women. Boron supplementation markedly elevated serum levels of 17-beta estradiol and testosterone; the elevation seemed more marked when dietary magnesium was low. These findings suggest that boron supplementation prevents calcium loss and bone demineralization.

17. F. H. Nielsen et al., "Boron Enhances and Mimics Some Effects of Estrogen Therapy in Postmenopausal Women," *Journal of Trace Elements in Experimental Medicine* 5 (1992): pp. 237-46.

18. F. H. Nielsen, "Facts and Fallacies About Boron," *Nutrition Today* (May/June 1992): pp. 6-12.

19. N. R. Calhoun, J. C. Smith, Jr., and K. L. Becker, "The Effects of Zinc on Ectopic Bone Formation," *Oral Surgery* 39 (1975): pp. 698-706.

20. M. Yamaguchi and T. Sakashita, "Enhancement of Vitamin D_3 Effect on Bone Metabolism in Weanling Rats Orally Administered Zinc Sulfate," *Acta Endocrinologica* 111 (1986): pp. 285-88.

21. O. S. Atik, "Zinc and Senile Osteoporosis," *Journal of the American Geriatrics Society* 31 (1983): pp. 790-91.

22. L. Frithiof et al., "The Relationship between Marginal Bone Loss and Serum Zinc Levels," *Acta Medica Scandinavica* 207 (1980): pp. 67-70.

23. R.H. Follis Jr. et al., "Studies on Copper Metabolism. XVIII. Skeletal Changes Associated with Copper Deficiency in Swine," *Bulletin of Johns Hopkins Hospitals* 97 (1955): pp. 405-09.

24. R. T. Smith et al., "Mechanical Properties of Bone from Copper Deficient Rats Fed Starch or Fructose," *Federation Proceedings* 44 (1985): p. 541.

25. E. M. Carlisle, "Silicon Localization and Calcification in Developing Bone," *Federation Proceedings* 28 (1969): p. 374.

26. L. Strause and P. Saltman, "Biochemical Changes in Rat Skeleton Following Long-Term Dietary Manganese and Copper Deficiencies," *Federation Proceedings* 44 (1985): p. 752.

27. P. D. Saltman and L. G. Strause, "The Role of Trace Minerals in Osteoporosis," *Journal of the American College of Nutrition* 12, no. 4 (1993): pp. 384-89.

Review article confirms the importance of trace minerals manganese, zinc and copper in studies of spinal bone mineral density in postmenopausal women.

28. A. R. Gaby, *Preventing and Reversing Osteoporosis* (Rockland, CA: Prima, 1994): p. 86.

29. L. E. Brattstrom et al., "Folic Acid—An Innocuous Means to Reduce Plasma Homocysteine," *Scandinavian Journal of Clinical and Laboratory Investigation* 48 (1988): pp. 215-21.

30. M. M. Nelson, W. R. Lyons, & H. M. Evans, "Maintenance of Pregnancy in Pyridoxine-Deficient Rats When Injected with Estrone and Progesterone," *Endocrinology* 48 (1951): pp. 726-32.

31. A. R. Gaby, *Preventing and Reversing Osteoporosis* (Rockland, CA: Prima, 1994): pp. 72-73.

32. Ibid., p. 96.

33. Z. R. Kime, *Sunlight* (Penryn, CA: World Health Publications, 1980): p. 153.

34. A. R. Gaby, *Preventing and Reversing Osteoporosis* (Rockland, CA: Prima, 1994): pp. 21-28.

35. O. Epstein, Y. Kato, R. Dick, & S. Sherlock, "Vitamin D, Hydroxyapatite, and Calcium Gluconate in Treatment of Cortical Bone Thinning in Postmenopausal Women with Primary Biliary Cirrhosis," *American Journal of Clinical Nutrition* 36 (Sept. 1982): pp. 426-30.

36. A. St. J. Dixon, "Non-Hormonal Treatment of Osteoporosis," *British Medical Journal* 286, no. 6370 (March 26, 1983): pp. 999-1000.
    With microcrystalline hydroxyapatite bone loss was halted and bone density improved.

37. *Medical Tribune* (July 22, 1993): p. 1, cited by R. A. Anderson in preconference workshop, American Holistic Medical Association Conference, Feb. 13-15, 1994, Seattle, WA.
    Of 31 women taking 250-750 mg magnesium daily for two years, 75% achieved bone mineral density increases of 1-8%. 17 women refusing the supplement had bone mineral losses of 1-3%.

38. F. H. Nielsen, C. D. Hunt, L. M. Mullen, & J. R. Hunt, *Effect of Dietary Boron on Mineral, Estrogen and Testosterone Metabolism in Postmenopausal Women* (Grand Forks, ND: U. S. Department of Agriculture, Agricultural Research Service, Grand Forks Human Nutrition Research Center): pp. 394-97.

39. A. R. Gaby, *Preventing and Reversing Osteoporosis* (Rockland, CA: Prima, 1994): pp. 41-42.

40. Ibid., p. 43.

41. G. P. Dalsky et al., "Weight-Bearing Exercise Training and Lumbar Bone Mineral Content in Postmenopausal Women," *Annals of Internal Medicine* 108, no. 6 (June 1988): pp. 824-28.
    A 6.1% increase in bone mass occurred in 35 women engaged in more than 50 minutes of exercise at 70-90% of VO_2 max three times a week for 22 months (walking, jogging, stair climbing) compared to a sedentary control group who experienced further losses in bone mass (-1.4%).

42. R. M. Neer et al., "Stimulation by Artificial Lighting of Calcium Absorption in Elderly Human Subjects," *Nature* 229 (Jan. 22, 1971): pp. 255-57.

43. R. Wurtman, quoted in H. Hellman, "Guiding Light," *Psychology Today* (April 1982), p. 27.

44. J. R. Lee, "Successful Menopausal Osteoporosis Treatment: Restoring Osteoclast/Osteoblast Equilibrium," (unpublished); and J. R. Lee, "Osteoporosis Reversal with Transdermal Progesterone" (letter), *Lancet* 336, no. 8726 (Nov. 24, 1990): p. 1327.

45. J. R. Lee, "Osteoporosis Reversal: The Role of Progesterone," *International Clinical Nutrition Review* 10, no. 3 (July 1990): pp. 386-91.

46. J. R. Lee, *Natural Progesterone: Multiple Roles of a Remarkable Hormone* (Sebastopol, CA: BLL, 1993).

47. A. R. Gaby, *Preventing and Reversing Osteoporosis* (Rockland, CA: Prima, 1994): p. 15.

48. C. W. Bales, "Nutritional Aspects of Osteoporosis: Recommendations for the Elderly at Risk," *Annual Review of Gerontology and Geriatrics* 9 (1989): pp. 7-34 (For caffeine, see p. 22).

 The amount of caffeine in one 10 oz. mug of coffee (150 mg) has been estimated to increase urinary calcium [excretion] by about 16 mg per day, equivalent to an increased calcium need of 60-100 mg when allowance is made for absorptive efficiency.

49. A. R. Gaby, *Preventing and Reversing Osteoporosis* (Rockland, CA: Prima, 1994): p. 12.

50. Ibid., p. 15.

51. M. Hernandez-Avila et al., "Caffeine, Moderate Alcohol Intake, and Risk of Fractures of the Hip and Forearm in Middle-Aged Women," *American Journal of Clinical Nutrition* 54 (1991): pp. 157-63.

52. K. A. Hollenbach, E. Barrett-Connor, S. L. Edelstein, & T. Holbrook, "Cigarette Smoking and Bone Mineral Density in Older Men and Women," *American Journal of Public Health* 83, no. 9 (Sep. 1993): pp. 1265-70.

53. *International Clinical Nutrition Review* 10 (July 1990): pp. 384-91, cited by R. A. Anderson in Preconference Workshop, American Holistic Medical Association Conference, Feb. 13-15, 1994, Seattle, WA.

 With a strong vitamin and mineral regimen, estrogen and progesterone, and exercise, no carbonated beverages, limited alcohol and a healthy diet, spontaneous osteoporotic fractures in 100 postmenopausal women were reduced to zero. There was an accompanying significant improvement in bone density over the treatment period of three years, stabilizing at the level of a healthy thirty-five year old.

54. A. R. Gaby, *Preventing and Reversing Osteoporosis* (Rockland, CA: Prima, 1994).

55. H. S. Hettiarachchy, S. S. S. Kantha, & S. M. X. Corea, "The Effect of Oral Contraceptive Therapy and of Pregnancy on Serum Folate Levels of Rural Sri Lankan Women," *British Journal of Nutrition* 50, no. 3 (Nov 1983): pp. 495-501.

 Folate levels dropped during pregnancy and during the use of birth control pills. After taking pills for more than 12 months, there was an even greater drop in serum folate.

56. C. E. Butterworth Jr. et al., "Improvement in Cervical Dysplasia Associated with Folic Acid Therapy in Users of Oral Contraceptives," *American Journal of Clinical Nutrition* 35 (Jan. 1982): pp. 73-82.

CHAPTER 11. WHAT ABOUT PROGESTERONE?

1. K. Dalton, *Once a Month* (4th ed.) (Claremont, CA: Hunter House, 1990).

2. P. J. Schmidt et al., "Lack of Effect of Induced Menses on Symptoms in Women with Premenstrual Syndrome," *New England Journal of Medicine* 324, no. 17 (Apr. 25, 1991): pp. 1174-79.

3. Personal conversations with Dr. Katharina Dalton in Aug. 1987.

4. K. Dalton, *Once a Month* (4th ed.) (Claremont, CA: Hunter House, 1990): p. 148.

5. C. R. Mabray et al., "Treatment of Common Gynecologic-Endocrinologic Symptoms by Allergy Management Procedures," *Obstetrics and Gynecology* 59, no. 5 (May 1982): pp. 560-64.

A protocol for provocative neutralization and treatment of PMS homeopathically with progesterone (.000000128 mg to .5 mg of aqueous progesterone subdermally) often produced "startlingly rapid and effective" clearing of symptoms.

CHAPTER 12. SLEEP

1. J. C. Friedrich, *The Pre-Menstrual Solution: How to Tame the Shrew in You* (San Jose, CA: Arrow, 1987).
2. "Amino Acids: A Link to PMS?" *PMS Access* (March/April 1986): pp. 1-2.
3. *Medical Tribune* (July 22, 1993): p. 15, cited by R. A. Anderson in Preconference Workshop, American Holistic Medical Association Conference, Feb. 13-15, 1994, Seattle, WA.

39 healthy elderly volunteers with insomnia given 2 mg of melatonin reduced their mean sleep onset delay from 40 minutes to 15 minutes.
4. W. Pierpaoli and W. Regelson, "Pineal Control of Aging: Effect of Melatonin and Pineal Grafting on Aging Mice," *Proceedings of the National Academy of Sciences USA* 91 (Jan. 1994): pp. 787-91.

Volunteers went to sleep in 5-6 minutes with melatonin vs 25 minutes on placebo. Subjects on melatonin also tended to sleep about twice as long as those on placebo. Other studies have shown that older people, who often suffer from insomnia, have far less melatonin in their bodies than young people.
5. R. Kotulak, "Blood Test May Identify Suicide-Prone People," *Chicago Tribune* (May 14, 1987): sec. 1, p. 4.

"The test, which measures levels of an important brain chemical called serotonin, has been found to accurately identify patients who suffered from depression and who tended toward suicidal behavior. [Dr. J. J. Mann, a Cornell Univ. psychiatrist, said that] low levels of the brain chemical have been associated with violent or aggressive behavior....The blood test measures prolactin levels, with low levels indicating low levels of serotonin in the brain. The evidence so far shows that low prolactin levels are associated with impulsivity, aggression and suicidal behavior."
6. R. J. Reiter, "The Pineal Gland: An Important Link to the Environment," *News in Physiological Sciences* 1 (Dec. 1986): pp. 202-5.
7. P. L. Delgado et al., "Serotonin Function and the Mechanism of Antidepressant Action," *Archives of General Psychiatry* 47 (May 1990): pp. 411-18.

Brain serotonin content is dependent on plasma levels of the essential amino acid tryptophan....Free plasma tryptophan level was negatively correlated with depression score during acute tryptophan depletion. The therapeutic effects of some antidepressant drugs may be dependent on serotonin availability.
8. A. J. Lewy and R. L. Sack, "Biological Rhythms and Behavior in Humans: The Effects of Light," ed. L Dennerstein and I. Fraser, *Hormones and Behaviour: Proceedings of the 8th International Congress of the International Society of Psychosomatic Obstetrics and Gynaecology*, Melbourne, Mar. 10-14, 1986, (Amsterdam: Excerpta Medica): p. 489.

All studies to date, which are small in number, have shown reduced melatonin plasma concentrations in depression.

9. J. Franklin, *Molecules of the Mind* (New York: Dell, 1987).

10. W. Dement, *The Sleepwatchers* (Stanford, CA: Stanford Alumni Assoc., 1992): p. 49.

11. A. J. Rapkin et al., "Whole-Blood Serotonin in Premenstrual Syndrome," *Obstetrics and Gynecology* 70, no. 4 (Oct. 1987): pp. 533-37.

12. J. FF. Watts, W. R. Butt, R. L. Edwards, & G. Holder, "Hormonal Studies in Women with Premenstrual Tension," *British Journal of Obstetrics and Gynaecology* 92 (March 1985): pp. 27-55.
Ovulation may occur 16-17 days before menstruation.

13. J. G. Lindsley, E. L. Hartmann, & W. Mitchell, "Selectivity in Response to L-Tryptophan Among Insomniac Subjects: A Preliminary Report," *Sleep* 6, no. 3 (1983): pp. 247-56.
Tryptophan was particularly successful in the "multiple awakening" group. "Single interruption" and "dozer" categories did not respond.

14. S. N. Young, "The Clinical Psychopharmacology of Tryptophan," ed. R. J. Wurtman and J. J. Wurtman, *Nutrition and the Brain* (New York: Raven Press, 1986): pp. 49-88.

15. E. Edelson, "Nutrition and the Brain," in *Encyclopedia of Psychoactive Drugs*, Series 2 (New York: Chelsea House, 1988): p. 55.

16. Ibid., p. 63.

17. R. J. Wurtman and J. D. Fernstrom, "Control of Brain Neurotransmitter Synthesis by Precursor Availability and Nutritional State," *Biochemical Pharmacology* 25, no. 15, pt. 2 (Aug. 1976): pp. 1691-96.
Sucrose ingestion can significantly elevate brain tryptophan and serotonin levels as well. The resulting shifts in serotonin-transmitter concentrations then have the potential for affecting mood, memory, intellectual function, and behavior.

18. N. J. Greenberger and K. J. Isselbacher, "Disorders of Absorption," ed. Braunwald et al., *Harrison's Principles of Internal Medicine,* 11th ed. (New York: McGraw-Hill, 1987): pp. 1260-76.
Neutral amino acids seem to share a common carrier mechanism, thus amino acids such as tryptophan and alanine show competitive inhibition. (p. 1261).

19. Ibid.

20. R. Malmgren, A. Collins, & C. G. Nilsson, "Platelet Serotonin Uptake and Effects of Vitamin B_6-Treatment in Premenstrual Tension," *Neuropsychobiology* 18 (1987): pp. 83-88.

21. S. N. Young, G. Chouinard, & L. Annable, "Tryptophan in the Treatment of Depression," *Advances in Experimental Medicine and Biology* 133 (1981): pp. 727-37.

22. J. C. Friedrich, *The Pre-Menstrual Solution: How to Tame the Shrew in You* (San Jose, CA: Arrow, 1987): pp. 41-42.

23. C. Thompson, D. Stinson, & A. Smith, "Seasonal Affective Disorder and Season-Dependent Abnormalities of Melatonin Suppression by Light," *Lancet* 336, no. 8717 (Sept. 22, 1990): pp. 703-6.

24. "U.S. Bars Diet Supplement L-Tryptophan, Warns of Blood Disorder," *Chicago Tribune* (Mar. 23, 1990): p. 8.

25. L. Slutsker et al., "Eosinophilia-myalgia Syndrome Associated with Exposure to L-Tryptophan from a Single Manufacturer," *Journal of the American Medical Association* 264, no. 2 (July 11, 1990): pp. 213-17.

26. J. Duffy, "Eosinophilia-Myalgia Syndrome," editorial, *Mayo Clinic Proceedings* 67 (1992): pp. 1201-2.

    Reviews studies that identify two contaminants in tryptophan made by one Japanese pharmaceutical manufacturer as the cause of the outbreak of EMS.

27. A. N. Mayeno et al., "Characterization of 'Peak E,' a Novel Amino Acid Associated with Eosinophilia-Myalgia Syndrome," *Science* 250 (1990): pp. 1707-8.

28. R. M. Jaffe, "Eosinophilia-Myalgia Syndrome Caused by Contaminated Tryptophan," *International Journal of Biosocial Medical Research* 11, no. 2 (1989): 181-84.

29. R. L. Pollack, *The Pain-Free Tryptophan Diet: The Dietary and Natural Amino Acid Program that Helps You Say Good-Bye to Pain Forever* (New York: Warner Brothers, 1986).

30. J. D. Fernstrom and R. J. Wurtman, "Nutrition and the Brain," *Scientific American* 230, no. 2 (Feb. 1974): pp. 84-91.

    A carbohydrate-rich meal increased serotonin levels in the brain, thus potentially affecting mind and mood function.

31. M. Dahlitz et al., "Delayed Sleep Phase Syndrome Response to Melatonin," *Lancet* 337, no. 8750 (May 11, 1991): pp. 1121-24.

    In persons with severe sleep-onset delay, melatonin advanced the sleep onset by 82 minutes more than placebo. Total sleep was reduced by 34 minutes with melatonin.

32. P. D. Leathwood, F. Chauffard, E. Heck, & R. Munoz-Box, "Aqueous Extract of Valerian Root (*Valeriana officinalis L.*) Improves Sleep Quality in Man," *Pharmacology Biochemistry and Behavior* 17, no. 1 (July 1982): pp. 65-71.

    Significantly better sleep quality and decreased sleep latency [onset] were reported with Valeriana officinalis L. extract 400 mg. Night awakenings were not affected.

33. H. Dressing, D. Reimann, et al., "Insomnia: Are Valerian/Melissa Combination of Equal Value to Benzodiazepine?" *Therapiewoche* 42 (1992): 726-36. Reported by D. J. Brown, *Townsend Letter for Doctors* (Jan. 1994): p. 124.

    Valerian/melissa preparation showed an effect comparable to that of the benzodiazepine as well as an increase in deep sleep stages 3 and 4. No daytime sedation or rebound phenomena were observed. Also, no restriction of concentration or physical performance was observed in either the Concentration Performance Test or the Labyrinth Test.

34. O. Lindahl and L. Linwall, "Double Blind Study of a Valerian Preparation," *Pharmacology Biochemistry and Behavior* 32, no. 4 (April 1989): pp. 1065-66.

    On the Valerian (Natt) night 89% reported improved sleep and 44% reported perfect sleep, significantly better than placebo.

CHAPTER 13. THE LIGHT CONNECTION

1. L. H. Back, "Multidisciplinary PMS Assessment Form." Paper presented at the Dalton Society for PMS Research, Education, Diagnosis and Treatment, Oct. 1989, Oklahoma City, OK.

2. C. Thompson, D. Stinson, & A. Smith, "Seasonal Affective Disorder and Season-Dependent Abnormalities of Melatonin Suppression by Light," *Lancet* 336, no. 8717 (Sept. 22, 1990): pp. 703-6.

3. R. E. McGrath, B. Buckwald, & E. V. Resnick, "The Effect of L-Tryptophan on Seasonal Affective Disorder," *Journal of Clinical Psychiatry* 51, no. 4 (April 1990): pp. 162-63.

4. B. L. Parry et al., "Altered Waveform of Plasma Nocturnal Melatonin Secretion in Premenstrual Depression," *Archives of General Psychiatry* 47 (1991): pp. 1139-46.

5. B. L. Parry, N. Rosenthal, L. Tamarkin, & T. Wehr, "Treatment of a Patient with Seasonal Premenstrual Syndrome," *American Journal of Psychiatry* 144, no. 6 (June 1987): pp. 762-66.

6. A. J. Lewy and R. L. Sack, "Biological Rhythms and Behavior in Humans: The Effects of Light," ed. L. Dennerstein and I. Fraser, *Hormones and Behaviour: Proceedings of the 8th International Congress of the International Society of Psychosomatic Obstetrics and Gynaecology*, Melbourne, Mar. 10-14, 1986, (Amsterdam: Excerpta Medica): p. 478.

7. A. Toufexis, "Dark Days, Darker Spirits," *Time*, (Jan. 11, 1988): p. 66.
   "Child psychiatrist William Sonis of the University of Pennsylvania, who in a 1985 survey found that 6.5% of 1,000 students at a suburban Minneapolis high school had SAD, says that 'too often the symptoms are attributed to school-related issues, like the seventh- or tenth-grade slump.' Or they are ascribed to behavior problems. The most prevalent symptom among children is irritability," says Sonis. 'Kids said they picked fights and they didn't know why.' The clue that their problems are due to SAD: depression recurs year after year."

8. S. Gallagher, "Solar Power," *American Health* 10, no. 1 (Jan./Feb. 1991): pp. 35-43.

9. M. L. Rao et al., "The Influence of Phototherapy on Serotonin and Melatonin in Non-Seasonal Depression," *Pharmacopsychiatry* 23, no. 3 (May 1990): pp. 155-58.

10. C. Thompson, D. Stinson, & A. Smith, "Seasonal Affective Disorder and Season-Dependent Abnormalities of Melatonin Suppression by Light," *Lancet* 336, no. 8717 (Sept. 22, 1990): pp. 703-6.

11. D. A. Redburn and C. K. Mitchell, "Darkness Stimulates Rapid Synthesis and Release of Melatonin in Rat Retina," *Visual Neuroscience* 3 (1989): pp. 391-403.

12. J. I. Nurnberger et al., "Supersensitivity to Melatonin Suppression by Light in Young People at High Risk for Affective Disorder: A Preliminary Report," *Neuropsychopharmacology* 1, no. 3 (Sept. 1988): pp. 217-23.

13. F. Winton et al., "Effects of Light Treatment Upon Mood and Melatonin in Patients with Seasonal Affective Disorder," *Psychological Medicine* 19, no. 3 (1989): pp. 585-90.

14. A. J. Rapkin et al., "Whole Blood Serotonin in Premenstrual Syndrome," *Obstetrics and Gynecology* 70 (1987): pp. 533-37.

15. Z. R. Kime, *Sunlight* (Penryn, CA: World Health, 1980): p. 29.

16. *Local Climatological Data: Chicago, Denver, San Diego*, National Oceanic and Atmospheric Administration, U.S. Department of Commerce (Asheville, North Carolina: National Climatic Data Center, 1988).

17. *Comparative Climatic Data for the United States through 1988*, National Oceanic and Atmospheric Administration, U.S. Department of Commerce (Asheville, North Carolina: National Climatic Data Center, 1988).

18. J. Liberman, *Light: Medicine of the Future* (Santa Fe: Bear, 1991).

19. Personal correspondence with I. Esslemont, April 10, 1991.

20. N. Rosenthal, *Seasons of the Mind* (New York: Bantam, 1989): pp. 76-78.

21. S. D. Moore, "Here at Ward Five, They Help Swedes Lighten Up a Little," *Wall Street Journal Europe* X, no. 11 (Jan. 14-15, 1992): p. 1.

22. J. Liberman, *Light: Medicine of the Future* (Santa Fe: Bear, 1991): p. 61.

23. R. Moreines, *Light up Your Blues* (New York: Berkeley, 1989): p. 46.

24. N. Sunderaraj et al., "Seasonal Behavior of Human Menstrual Cycles: A Biometric Investigation," *Human Biology* 50, no. 1. (1978): p. 29.

25. F. A. Cook, "Some Physical Effects of Arctic Cold, Darkness, and Light," *Medical Record* 51 (1897): p. 835.

26. M. H. Smolensky, "Aspects of Human Chronopathology," ed. A. Reinberg and M. H. Smolensky, *Biological Rhythms and Medicine: Cellular, Metabolic, Physiopathologic, and Pharmacologic Aspects* (New York: Springer Verlag, 1983): pp. 137-39.
    Cites 13 studies.

27. E. M. Dewan, "On the Possibility of a Perfect Rhythm Method of Birth Control by Periodic Light Stimulation," *American Journal of Obstetrics and Gynecology* 99 (1967): pp. 1016-19.

28. E. M. Dewam, M. F. Menkin, and J. Rock, "Effect of Photic Stimulation on the Human Menstrual Cycle," *Photochemistry and Photobiology* 27 (1978): pp. 581-85.

29. L. Lacey, *Lunaception* (New York: Coward, McCann & Geoghegan, 1974): p. 117.

30. Personal communication with Henry Savage, fall 1994. Research headed by Dan Kripke, M.D., UCSD.

31. Personal communication with H. Lahmeyer, M.D., Dir., Dept. of Psychiatry, Northwestern Univ., Oct. 7, 1994.

32. B. L. Parry, N. E. Rosenthal, L. Tamarkin, & T. A. Wehr, "Treatment of a Patient with Seasonal Premenstrual Syndrome," *American Journal of Psychiatry* 144, no. 6 (June 1987): pp. 762-66.
    SAD and PMS have numerous common symptoms. Case history: Melatonin given to SAD patient resulted in significant improvement.

33. N. Rosenthal, *Seasons of the Mind* (New York: Bantam, 1989): p. 17.

34. J. N. Ott, *Health and Light* (Old Greenwich, CT: Devin-Adair, 1973).

35. Z. R. Kime, *Sunlight* (Penryn, CA: World Health Publications, 1980).

36. J. Liberman, *Light: Medicine of the Future* (Santa Fe: Bear, 1991).

37. J. S. Adams, T. L. Clemens, J. A. Parrish, & M. F. Holick, "Vitamin-D Synthesis and Metabolism after Ultraviolet Irradiation of Normal and Vitamin-D-Deficient Subject," *New England Journal of Medicine* 306, no. 12 (Mar. 25, 1982): pp. 722-25.

38. R. M. Neer et al., "Stimulation by Artificial Lighting of Calcium Absorption in Elderly Human Subjects," *Nature* 229 (Jan. 22, 1971): pp. 255-57.

39. F. A. Stevens, "The Bacteriocidal Properties of UV-Irradiated Lipids of the Skin," *Journal of Experimental Medicine* 65 (1937): p. 121.

40. V. Beral et al., "Malignant Melanoma and Exposure to Fluorescent Light at Work," *Lancet* 2, no. 8293 (Aug. 7, 1982): pp. 290-93.

41. Note: The following references (#42-61) are based on the research of Jacob Liberman, O.D., Ph.D., and are included his book *Light: Medicine of the Future* (Santa Fe: Bear, 1991): pp. 141-44. They are used with his permission:

42. M. F. Holick and M. B. Clark, "The Photobiogenesis and Metabolism and Vitamin D," *Federation Proceedings* 37 (1978): p. 2567.

43. M. F. Holick et al., "Advances in the Photobiology of Vitamin D-3," (Second Annual Scientific Meeting of the American Society for Bone and Mineral Research, Washington, D.C., U.S.A., June 16-17, 1980) *CALCIF Tissue International* 31, no. 1, p. 79.

44. M. F. Holick et al., "Photosynthesis of Previtamin D-3 in Human Skin and the Physiologic Consequences," *Science* 210 (Oct. 10, 1980): pp. 203-5.

45. M. F. Holick, J. A. MacLaughlin, and S. H. Doppelt, "Regulation of Cutaneous Previtamin D-3 Photosynthesis in Man: Skin Pigment Is Not An Essential Regulator," *Science* 211 (Feb. 6, 1981): pp. 590-93.

46. J. A. MacLaughlin, R. R. Anderson, and M. F. Holick, "Spectral Character of Sunlight Modulates Photosynthesis of Previtamin D-3 and Its Photoisomers in Human Skin," *Science* 216 (May 28, 1982): pp. 1001-3.

47. R. M. Neer et al., "Stimulation by Artificial Lighting of Calcium Absorption in Elderly Human Subjects," *Nature* 229 (Jan. 22, 1971): pp. 255-57.

48. J. R. Johnson, "The Effect of Carbon Arc Radiation on Blood Pressure and Cardiac Output," *American Journal of Physiology* 114 (1935): p. 594.

49. Ibid.

50. L. Lohmeier, "Let the Sun Shine In," *East West* (July 1986): pp. 36-39.

51. L. A. Kunitsina et al., "Therapeutic Action of Ultraviolet Irradiation in a Complex Treatment of Patients with Initial Cerebral Atherosclerosis," *Sovet Med* 33 (1970): p. 89.

52. V. A. Mikhailov, "Influence of Graduated Sunlight Baths on Patients with Coronary Athersoclerosis," *Sovet Med* 29 (1966): p. 76.

53. A. I. Pertsovskij et al., "Preventative Activity of Ultraviolet Rays on the Presence of Experimental Atherosclerosis," *Vop Kurort Fizioter* 36 (1971): p. 203.

54. R. Altschul and I. H. Herman, "Ultraviolet Irradiation and Cholesterol Metabolism; Seventh Annual Meeting of The American Society for the Study of Arteriosclerosis," *Circulation* 8 (1953): p. 438.

55. L. Lohmeier, "Let the Sun Shine In," *East West* (July 1986): pp. 36-39.

56. Ibid.

57. I. I. Belyayev et al., "Combined Use of Ultraviolet Radiation to Control Acute Respiratory Disease," *Vestn Akad Med Nauk SSSR* 3 (1975): p. 37.

58. N. M. Dantsig, "Ultraviolet Radiation," in Russian language book (Moscow: 1966).

59. A. P. Zabaluyeva, "General Immunological Reactivity of the Organism in Prophylactic Ultraviolet Irradiation of Children in Northern Regions," *Vestn Akad Med Nauk SSSR* 3 (1975): p. 23.

60. T. K. Das Gupta and J. Terz, "Influence of Pineal Gland on the Growth and Spread of Melanoma in the Hamster," *Cancer Research* 27 (1967): p. 1306.
61. W. Stumpf et al., *Brain Mind Bulletin* 15, no. 1 (Oct. 1989): p. 2.
62. R. Liebmann-Smith, "The Man Who Patented Sunlight," *American Health* (Dec. 1985): pp. 32-35.

CHAPTER 14 CANDIDA - OR WHY DO I STILL FEEL SO BAD?
1. C. O. Truss, *The Missing Diagnosis* (Birmingham, AL: Author, 1983).
2. W. G. Crook, *The Yeast Connection: A Medical Breakthrough* (Jackson, TN: Professional, 1984).
3. R. T. Golan, "Yeast Overgrowth." From the manuscript of *Optimal Wellness* (New York: Ballantine, publication pending 1995): p. 10.
4. W. G. Crook, "Depression Associated with *Candida Albicans* Infections" (letter to the editor), *Journal of the American Medical Association* 251, no. 22 (June 8, 1984): pp. 2928-29.
   Depression is a component of the symptomatic presentation of Candidiasis. As C. albicans overgrowth is treated, including the use of nystatin, the depression improves.
5. D. Feldman, Presentation to the Third Yeast-Human Interaction Symposium, San Francisco, March 29-31, 1985, sponsored by the International Health Foundation, Jackson, TN. In J. P. Trowbridge and M. Walker, *The Yeast Syndrome: How to Help Your Doctor Identify and Treat the Real Cause of Your Yeast-Related Illness* (New York: Bantam, 1986): pp. 60-62.
6. Ibid., p. 18.
7. I. Neuhauser and E. L. Gustus, "Successful Treatment of Intestinal Moniliasis with Fatty Acid-Resin Complex." *Archives of Internal Medicine* 93 (1954): pp. 53-60.
8. L. DeSchepper, *Candida* (Westlake, CA: LDS, 1986).
9. L. Chaitow, *Candida Albicans: Could Yeast Be Your Problem?* (Rochester, Vermont: Healing Arts, 1988): p. 71.
10. M. Adetumbi, G. T. Javor, & B. H. S. Lau, "*Allium sativum* (Garlic) Inhibits Lipid Synthesis by *Candida Albicans*," *Antimicrobial Agents and Chemotherapy* 30, no. 3 (Sept. 1986): pp. 499-501.
    Garlic (Allium sativum) as a dehydrated powder totally arrested the lipid synthesis of Candida albicans in vitro. Growth of the organism was inhibited and protein and nucleic acid synthesis were inhibited to the same degree.
11. S. Warshafsky, R. S. Kamer, and S. L. Sivak, "Effect of Garlic on Total Serum Cholesterol," *Annals of Internal Medicine* 119, no. 7 (Oct. 1, 1993): pp. 599-605.
12. J. Avorn et al., "Reduction of Bacteriuria and Pyuria After Ingestion of Cranberry Juice," *Journal of the American Medical Association* 271, no. 10 (Mar. 9, 1994): pp. 751-54.
13. L. Chaitow, *Candida Albicans: Could Yeast Be Your Problem?* (Rochester, Vermont: Healing Arts, 1988): pp. 69-70.
14. J. S. Schinfeld, "PMS and Candidiasis: Study Explores Possible Link," *Female Patient* 12, no. 7 (July 1987): pp. 66-74.
    A controlled study in which women with recalcitrant PMS and recurrent candidiasis were treated with a combination of medication and a yeast-elimination diet. Of 32 women, 15 went on a sucrose- and yeast-free diet

and oral nystatin. 10 of these had significant relief from premenstrual symptoms. The control group of 17 failed to show any change in symptoms.

15. P. Radetsky, "The Yeast Within," *Discover* (March 1994): pp. 45-49.
16. V. Glassburn, *Who Killed Candida?* (Brushton, NY: TEACH Service, 1991).
17. R. T. Golan, "Yeast Overgrowth." From the manuscript of *Optimal Wellness* (New York: Ballantine, publication pending 1995).
18. H. E. Hagglund, *Why Do I Feel So Bad (When the Doctor Says I'm OK?): Candida Albicans May Be the Answer* (Oklahoma City, OK: IED Press, 1984).
19. H. E. Hagglund, (Producer-Director). *Yeast Story* [videotape] (Norman, OK: Tele-Visits, n.d.).
20. S. Lorenzani, *Candida: A Twentieth-Century Disease* (New Canaan, CT: Keats, 1986).
21. J. P. Trowbridge and M. Walker, *The Yeast Syndrome: How to Help Your Doctor Identify and Treat the Real Cause of Your Yeast-Related Illness* (New York: Bantam, 1986).
22. D. Nolan, *Ending Fatigue and Depression* (Redmond, WA: James, McCormick, 1987).
23. W. G. Crook, *The Yeast Connection: A Medical Breakthrough* (Jackson, TN: Professional, 1984).
24. W. G. Crook, *The Yeast Connection and the Woman* (Jackson, TN: Professional, 1995).

Chapter 15. Candida Questionnaire

1. V. Glassburn, *Who Killed Candida?* (Brushton, NY: TEACH Service, 1991): pp. 34-36.

Chapter 16. Exercise

1. J. F. Steege and J. A. Blumenthal, "The Effects of Aerobic Exercise on Premenstrual Symptoms in Middle-Aged Women: A Preliminary Study," *Journal of Psychosomatic Research* 37, no. 2 (1993): pp. 127-33.
2. J. C. Prior et al., "Conditioning Exercise Decreases Premenstrual Symptoms: A Prospective, Controlled 6-Month Trial," *Fertility and Sterility* 47, no. 3 (Mar. 1987): pp. 402-8.
3. J. A. Blumenthal et al, "Stress Reactivity and Exercise Training in Premenopausal and Postmenopausal Women," *Health Psychology: The Official Journal of the Division of Health Psychology, American Psychological Association* 10, no. 6 (1991): pp. 384-91.
4. E. Kaufmann, "The New Rhythms of Fitness: The Shape of Workouts to Come," *American Health* (Dec. 1989): pp. 45-49.
5. S. K. Powers and E. T. Howley, *Exercise Physiology: Theory and Application to Fitness and Performance* (Dubuque, IA: Brown, 1990).
6. E. Kaufmann, "The New Rhythms of Fitness: The Shape of Workouts to Come," *American Health* (Dec. 1989): pp. 45-49.
7. M. Back, *Seven Half-Miles from Home: Notes of a Wind River Naturalist* (Boulder, CO: Johnson Books, 1985).
8. Z. R. Kime, *Sunlight* (Penryn, CA: World Health, 1980): pp. 33-47.

CHAPTER 17. STRESS

1. H. Benson with M. Z. Klipper, *The Relaxation Response* (New York: Avon, 1975).

2. J. Kabat-Zinn, *Full Catastrophe Living: Using the Wisdom of Your Body and Mind to Face Stress, Pain, and Illness* (New York: Delta, 1990).

3. F. Petty, G. L. Kramer, C. M. Gullion, & A. J. Rush, "Low Plasma Gamma-Aminobutyric Acid Levels in Male Patients with Depression," *Biological Psychiatry* 32 (1992): pp. 354-63.

CHAPTER 18. OTHER POSSIBLE CAUSES

1. W. Crook, *Are You Allergic: A Guide to Normal Living for Allergic Adults and Children* (Professional Books: Jackson, TN,1978).

2. N. S. Orenstein and S. L. Bingham, *Food Allergies: How to Tell if You Have Them, What to Do About Them if You Do* (New York: Perigee, 1987).

3. J. V. Wright, *Dr. Wright's Book of Nutritional Therapy* (Emmaus, PA: Rodale, 1985).

4. R. Buist, *Food Intolerance: What It Is and How to Cope with It* (Great Britain: Prism, 1984).

5. T. G. Randolph and R. W. Moss, *An Alternative Approach to Allergies: The New Field of Clinical Ecology Unravels the Environmental Causes of Mental and Physical Ills* (New York: Harper & Row, 1990 Revised Edition).

6. C. E. Bates, *Beyond Allergies: Relief from Persistent Hunger.* (Olympia, WA: Tsolum River, 1994).

7. Great Smokies Laboratory, 18A Regent Park Blvd., Asheville, NC 28806. Phone 800 522-4762 (U.S.); 800 833-5524 (Canada).

8. T. G. Randolph and R. W. Moss, *An Alternative Approach to Allergies: The New Field of Clinical Ecology Unravels the Environmental Causes of Mental and Physical Ills* (New York: Harper & Row, 1990 Revised Edition).

9. R. L. Siblerud, "The Relationship between Mercury from Dental Amalgam and Mental Health," *American Journal of Psychotherapy* 43, no. 4 (Oct. 1989): pp. 575-87.

    PMS, fatigue, poor memory, and stress were significantly improved following removal of mercury fillings.

10. S. Ziff, *Silver Dental Fillings: The Toxic Time Bomb* (New York: Aurora, 1984).

11. Dental Amalgam Mercury Syndrome (DAMS), Inc., 6025 Osuna Blvd. NE, Suite B, Albuquerque, NM 87109-2523. Phone 505 888-0111, Fax 505 888-4554.

12. R. T. Golan, "Adrenal Exhaustion." From the manuscript *Optimal Wellness* (New York: Ballantine, publication pending 1995).

13. E. Bass and L. Davis, *The Courage to Heal: A Guide for Women Survivors of Child Sexual Abuse.* (New York: Harper Perennial, 1988, rev. 1992).

14. L. Davis, *The Courage to Heal Workbook: For Women and Men Survivors of Child Sexual Abuse* (New York: Harper & Row, 1990).

CHAPTER 19. PUTTING THE PUZZLE TOGETHER

1. P. Airola, *Hypoglycemia: A Better Approach* (Phoenix: Health Plus, 1977).

APPENDIX A. TAKING ACTION

1. M. H. Messer, R. Coronado-Bogdaniak, & L. J. Dillon, *Managing Anger: A Handbook of Proven Techniques* (Chicago: Cope, 1993).
2. H. G. Lerner, *The Dance of Anger* (New York: Harper & Row, 1985).

APPENDIX C. REFERENCE APPENDIX

1. *The Kellogg Report: The Impact of Nutrition, Environment and Lifestyle on the Health of Americans* (Annandale-on-Hudson, New York: The Institute of Health Policy and Practice of The Bard College Center, 1989), quotes Dr. Wodicka from Michael F. Jacobson, *Nutrition Scorecard: Your Guide to Better Eating*, 1975:78, p. 158.
2. M. Brin, "Red Cell Transketolase as an Indicator of Nutritional Deficiency," *American Journal of Clinical Nutrition* 33 (Feb. 1980): pp.169-71.

ABOUT THE AUTHOR

Linaya Hahn started researching PMS in the early 1980s when she developed severe PMS herself. She soon discovered that she was not the only woman seeking information about PMS.

Since then, she has read research from and worked with top PMS researchers and practitioners from around the world. After successfully controlling her own PMS, she found herself teaching other women how to reverse their PMS. Ms. Hahn was a PMS counselor and manager of a women's health center for several years before starting the PMS Holistic Center in 1985.

Ms. Hahn has become a recognized expert in the field of PMS care. She is a Founding Member of the Dalton Society, the international organization for PMS research, education, diagnosis, and treatment. Ms. Hahn is also a member of the International and American Association of Clinical Nutritionists and the American Holistic Medical Association. She is a published author in scientific journals and has addressed international PMS symposia and a conference of the American College of Obstetricians and Gynecologists. She holds a magna cum laude B.A. from Washburn University and is pursuing a graduate degree combining psychology, nutrition, and light.

She has also played a prominent role in increasing popular knowledge about PMS. She has been interviewed for several major publications, including feature articles in *Seventeen* and the *Chicago Tribune*, and has appeared on *The Oprah Show.*

Prior to her career as a PMS researcher/educator, Linaya raised two sons (and two dogs). She served as president of her local school board and as president of her branch of the American Association of University Women.

Ms. Hahn is available for speeches and phone consultations. Please contact the PMS Holistic Center at 708 520-3822 for available times and fees.

ABOUT THE ARTIST

Art Henrikson is a political cartoonist for Paddock Publications in suburban Chicago. His work is in permanent collections in the Library of Congress, Archives of American Art, the State Historical Society of Missouri, and Ohio State University. His art has been exhibited at the Art Institute of Chicago, the White House, and in major cities across the country and abroad. He has received numerous awards, including nine from the Freedom Foundation. He also medaled in the medical Caricature Exhibit Sessions in Verona, Italy. His work has enlightened several books.

Henrikson is a graduate of Northwestern University, where he was staff cartoonist for the Daily Northwestern and the school humor magazine. He also studied cartooning at the Chicago Academy of Fine Arts. He is a member of the Association of American Editorial Cartoonists and of Sigma Delta Chi, the Society of Professional Journalists. He lives in suburban Chicago, where he and his wife have raised three daughters. (No wonder he's interested in PMS control!) We are honored that he has contributed to this book.

INDEX

Traditional Healthy
  Mediterranean Diet, 50-51
Truss, Orian, 96
Tryptophan, 77-78
  contamination as cause for
  EMS, 79
  conversion to serotonin, 78-79
  food sources for, 80
Tuberculosis, and ultraviolet light
  in treating, 91

Ultraviolet light, 89-91
  UV-A, 89, 93
  UV-B, 89-90, 93
  UV-C, 90
Unsuspected Illness (Barnes), 42
Urinary tract infections, 99, 102

Vaginal infection, 95
  See Yeast infection
Vaginal itching or burning as
  PMS, 26
Vaginal progesterone
  suppositories, 71
Vaginal secretions, 8, 9
Vaginitis, Candida as cause of, 98
Valerian root as sleep aid, 80-81
Visible light, 89
Vitamin A, 61
  as beta carotene, 61
Vitamin B_6
  effects of, 64
  in PMS, 62, 78
Vitamin C
  effects of, 64
  RDA recommendations on, 60
Vitamin D_3
  in bone formation, 66
  effects of, 64
  UV-B in simulating production
  of, 89
Vitamin K, effects of, 64

Vitamins
  in building up immune system,
  100-1
  importance of, 147
  lack of, as cause of PMS, 59-68
  stages of deficiencies in, 147

Weight gain as PMS, 26
Weight loss, and ultraviolet light,
  91
Weight training, effect of, on
  PMS, 113
Withdrawal from others, as PMS,
  26
Work, absence from, as PMS, 17
Wright, Jonathan, 128-29
Wright-Gaby Nutrition
  Foundation, 42

Yeast Connection, The (Crook),
  96-97
Yeast infection, 97, 99
  See Vaginitis
Yogurt in controlling Candida,
  101

Ziff, Sam, 130
Zinc, effects of, 64

ORDER FORM

We have included an order form because it would be a disservice to give you information on how to control PMS without giving you a place to obtain the products you need. Products and prices change over time, so it is impractical to include a complete product and price list. We will add new items as our research and your requests indicate. We pledge to offer the highest quality products at the lowest possible prices. We have included some product information in the Resource Appendix (page 148). For up-to-date information, or to order by telephone, call 800 520-3822.

Product:_____Quantity _____

_____Quantity _____

_____Quantity _____

Ordered by:

Name _____

Address _____

City _____

State/Province _____ Zip/Postal Code _____

Daytime Phone (_____) _____

Ship to (if different from above):

Name _____

Address _____

City _____State____Zip _____

Method of Payment

☐ VISA   ☐ MasterCard   ☐ Check or Money Order

Card Number _____ Exp. Date _____

Name on card _____

Signature _____